The Psychoanalytic Couch

The Psychoanalytic Couch offers a comprehensive overview and a poetic rethinking of the psychoanalytic couch.

Part I presents an extensive study of how the couch has been implicitly or explicitly theorised by major figures in the field, including Freud, Ferenczi, Winnicott, Bion, Bollas, Ogden, Green, and Lacan, by extracting, organising, and developing their dispersed contributions on the subject. Part II moves into the poetic and etymological realm of the word *diwan*, tracing its roots to Persian and Arabic traditions. Krüger develops an original model for clinical listening and intervention, where the "cloud state" plays an important role in analytic technique. Concepts such as condensation (*Verdichtung*), symbolic vesture and the structuring of psychic regions are reinterpreted through this prism, offering a new way to conceptualize transference and analytic presence. The book fulfils a significant gap in psychoanalytic theory and training by elevating a central yet neglected clinical element to conceptual prominence.

The Psychoanalytic Couch will be essential reading for psychoanalysts in practice and in training, and for readers interested in the intersections between psychoanalysis, art and literature.

Lucas Krüger is a psychoanalyst, writer, musician, translator and editor based in Brazil. He is the author of books on psychoanalysis, poetry and children's literature, and has edited over 70 titles. His work bridges psychoanalysis and the arts while bringing the field's historical legacy into dialogue with contemporary practice, raising new questions for clinical reflection.

The Psychoanalytic Couch

Listening Perspectives and the Poetics of Psychoanalysis

Lucas Krüger

Routledge
Taylor & Francis Group
LONDON AND NEW YORK

Designed cover image: Drawing and digital artwork by Lucas Krüger.

First published in English 2026
by Routledge
4 Park Square, Milton Park, Abingdon, Oxon OX14 4RN

and by Routledge
605 Third Avenue, New York, NY 10158

Routledge is an imprint of the Taylor & Francis Group, an informa business

First published in Portuguese by Editora Blucher and Artes & Ecos. Por que o divã? Perspectivas de escuta e a poética da psicanálise (2023).

British Library Cataloguing-in-Publication Data
A catalogue record for this book is available from the British Library

ISBN: 978-1-041-15795-3 (hbk)
ISBN: 978-1-041-15793-9 (pbk)
ISBN: 978-1-003-68121-2 (ebk)

DOI: 10.4324/9781003681212

Typeset in Times New Roman
by SPi Technologies India Pvt Ltd (Straive)

For Marília and Inácio,
for all their love and patience during the writing process.

Contents

About the author

Lucas Krüger is a Brazilian psychoanalyst, a full member of the Sigmund Freud Psychoanalytic Association in Porto Alegre and a member of the Brazilian Group for Sándor Ferenczi Studies. He is the author of *Why the Couch? Listening Perspectives and the Poetics of Psychoanalysis* (2023) and *Interlocutions on the Border between Psychoanalysis and Art* (2017). He has also published poetry books, including *The Dream of the Comma* (2015) and *Homage to the* Cloud (2017), as well as the children's book *The Rooster's Bald Spot* (2018). In addition, he has taken part in several musical projects. As a translator, he has contributed to the publication of *Arctic Poems* by Vicente Huidobro (2018), *Dreams, Melodies and Symptoms* by Sándor Ferenczi (2019), and *Dream and Myth: A Study on the Psychology of Peoples* by Karl Abraham (2020). He directs two editorial series – *Ferenczi: Translations from the Original* (since 2025) and *Psychoanalytic Writing* (since 2019) – which bring together contemporary essays and new translations of classic authors such as Karl Abraham, Lou Andreas-Salomé, Sabina Spielrein, Otto Gross, Ernst Simmel, Margarete Hilferding and Karen Horney. He is the founder and editor of Artes & Ecos, a publishing house dedicated to psychoanalysis, poetry and art, through which he has overseen the publication of more than 70 titles.

On the couch/*divã/divan/diván/diwan*

Key considerations regarding the English edition

Although in English the piece of furniture used technically by psychoanalysts is commonly referred to as a *couch* – the same term used for a sofa – other languages maintain clearer distinctions. For example, in Portuguese, *divã* refers specifically to the furniture used in the analytic setting, while *sofá* denotes a generic domestic item. In Spanish, the term *diván* is used, and in French, *divan*, both retaining this clinical specificity.

In this English edition, the term *couch* will be used, in accordance with standard usage in psychoanalytic literature, although the conceptual distinction between *couch* and *divã/divan/diván* remains significant. Whenever the word *couch* appears in this edition, the reader should bear in mind that, in the original, the word written was *divã*.

This book was originally written in Portuguese. All foreign texts cited were first translated into that language, and some of the discussions I propose – though not many – inevitably evoke dialogues primarily directed toward Brazilian psychoanalysts. I have preferred to preserve the book as it was published in its first edition, bearing in mind that translations in themselves cannot reproduce the same linguistic effects – a prime example being the entire theoretical construction based on the term *divã/diván/divan/diwan*, which diverges from the Anglophone usage, accustomed to calling this psychoanalytic piece of furniture a *couch*.

The etymology and symbolic dimensions of the term (*diwan*) will be explored in greater depth in Part II of this book. In any case, all these terms as used by psychoanalysts refer to the same piece of furniture. In the 1913 text *On Beginning the Treatment*, when addressing the item as a remnant of the hypnotic method, Freud refers to it as a *Ruhebett* – literally, a "resting bed."

Beyond these important technical remarks, I would also like to express my deep gratitude to my editor, Susannah Frearson, for her attentive guidance and commitment throughout the process that has culminated in this English edition.

Lucas Krüger

Preface

The unpredictable couch

Daniel Kupermann

Surprise. That's the word I found to express my experience of reading *The Psychoanalytic Couch: Listening Perspectives and the Poetics of Psychoanalysis* by Lucas Krüger. My eyes, accustomed to – and sometimes tired of – reading hundreds of books, dissertations, theses and articles published in periodicals on psychoanalysis, widened at many passages and landscapes, curious to know the paths that would be taken by this erudite, creative and provocative writing, focused on the object that has become the greatest symbol of psychoanalysis: the couch.

Couch (*divã/divan*). To non-psychoanalysts, the word sounds like something from a grandmother. *Divans* are rarely found as part of the furniture in privileged homes in the West these days, perhaps because the couch is associated with reading, resting, contemplating, daydreaming, imagination and dreaming. And in the society of tiredness, there is little room for these useless activities, according to the performance imperative to which we are subjected.

If the couch (*divã/divan*) remains part of the psychoanalytic furniture, that says a lot about what psychoanalysis is. Credit to Freud and his followers, who seem to insist on maintaining a very special place, a *topic* in our cultural environment, which imposes itself as a *reserve* – in the sense we say ecological reserve – for the exercise of listening and singular poetics, which often seem to be heading towards extinction.

It was a surprise to follow the rich developments undertaken by Lucas Krüger from the etymology of the term couch/divan, which derives from *diwan*, in its Persian and Turko-Ottoman forms. The first meaning refers to poetics, either to the writer himself or to a collection of poetry. The second refers to the spatial concept of the meeting room where important issues were decided by the sultans. In addition to these meanings, there is also the derivation *aduana* – the sound of which reveals its etymology, that is to say, control of the entry and exit of goods transported from one place to another. One should remember that, in German, the word *Übertragung*, used by Freud as a clinical concept, translated as transference, also means transport from one place to another. In this case, the transport of affections referring to existential experiences, whether traumatic or vitalising, from the analysand's unconscious memory system to the figure of the psychoanalyst, making the past of the person lying on the couch present.

Let there be no mistake. The aim of *The Psychoanalytic Couch: Listening Perspectives and the Poetics of Psychoanalysis* is not only to awaken us to the plethora of meanings embedded in the most characteristic furniture of psychoanalysis offices, but to sensitise us to the specificity of psychoanalytic practice itself, adopting the couch as its greatest metaphor.

Procrustes' couch/divan

Metaphors are antidotes to sterilising dogmatism. They take letters and words and turn upside down, perpetuating their polysemy. In Krüger's book, the couch is taken as the preliminary metaphor for a succession of conceptual metaphors that favour a living transmission of psychoanalytic practice.

Throughout its history, psychoanalysis has built veritable couches of Procrustes, in the form of institutes and schools dedicated to training analysts, according to the prevailing thinking in these spaces – to the point where an author like Michael Balint states that the great challenge for the psychoanalyst in training would be to escape from the requirement of obedience imposed on them, be it through institutional interference in "didactic" analyses, or the compulsory adoption of a single language to testify to the analytic experience, engendering a mere echolalia of the masters' words and uncritical adherence to current theories.

There is an implicit proposition in Lucas Krüger's book: the psychoanalyst, in his or her training process, should constitute a theoretical-clinical *self* that is attuned to his or her style and capable of encounters and disagreements with other analysts' theoretical-clinical *selves*. The development of psychoanalytic thought depends on these encounters and disagreements. In order to constitute a theoretical-clinical *self*, however, it would be necessary to introject the couch, constituting something close to what André Green called the internal frame, which would also allow us to take our inner couch to any and all spaces where psychoanalysis is called upon in its listening and poetics.

Thus, we find a mobile couch (not to miss the pun), nomadic in the transferential sense, capable of being taken to meet every psychic suffering, whether in the psychoanalyst's office, in the hospital, in schools, on the streets or on computer screens and mobile phones, as the universalised remote consultations imposed on us during the pandemic. A couch characterised, unlike the one covered with Freud's Persian rugs, by the lightness of a cloud that, walking, welcomes the flight of the imagination that has escaped from the stone statue, provoked by Medusa's terrifying gaze.[1]

The couch made by Lucas Krüger reminds us of the "cloud state", offering a real antidote to the tendency to create Procrustean couches in the various places where psychoanalysis is transmitted.

Look up

The cloud is, in fact, the inspiring muse of the author's conceptualisation of psychoanalytic poetics, who, it should be noted, published a book of poetry a few years ago entitled *Homage to the Cloud*. A surprise for those unversed in poetry, but an obvious connection in hindsight: the cloud is a very present inspiration in the field of poetry, from Goethe to Carlos Drummond de Andrade.

It couldn't be any different. The *formless* matter of which clouds are made offers itself, in the physical world, as the most eloquent image of a malleable medium necessary for the poet to believe in his power to create worlds. Clouds, with their play of moving forms, are, for the imagination of those who know how to look upwards, like letters capable of composing the words we need to celebrate our short and unpredictable existence. Ludwig Tieck, quoted in this book, writes: "Great elephant! Stretch out your trunk, / says the child to the stretching cloud / And the cloud obeys". I have no doubt that the first poet was the one who raised his eyes to the sky and, in tune with the play of the clouds, was able to sublimate the power of his voice into magical words.

It may be that Freud was actually a tobacco addict and was therefore always smoking during his sessions with his patients. However, after reading *The Psychoanalytic Couch*, I imagine that, alongside his love for the scent of burning tobacco and for the effect of nicotine in his blood, Freud developed the psychoanalytic method because he was transported into a "cloud state", inspired by the whirls of smoke rising from the tip of his cigar and from that exhaled from his lips.

By proposing that the analysand lie on the couch, the analyst invites them to turn their gaze away from their face and to look upward, freeing them from the play of demands for love, recognition and power that characterise our social relations.

Looking upwards reproduces the gesture of the primordial poet, fostering a regression to the primary processes of thought characteristic of the dream – the royal road to the poetics of the unconscious, according to Freud. In this "cloud state", to which the analysand is transported, it becomes possible to work through the pain, transmute the ghosts referred to in unconscious childhood imagery, the emergence of the omnipotent gesture of the child that resides in each one of us, favouring the creation of new forms of being, which come to inhabit the analytic space made into a cloud, as if they were levitating Chagall figures, with which the analysand can compose their stylistics of existence.

Customs/*aduana*

The conceptual metaphor "cloud state" proposed by Krüger is a testimony, in his own name, about the core of the psychoanalytic experience, defined as listening and poetics. Listening to the analysand's traumatic nuclei, as well as their desire to meet the vitalising Other, enunciated through different modes of expression, whether through words, silence or play. Listening, on the part of the analyst, to the way in which they are themselves affected in the exercise of their craft. Poetics as the possible creation, through the affective encounter, capable of affecting both partners in this adventure called psychoanalysis.

One of our greatest epistemological difficulties is finding a conceptual language capable of illustrating the space where subjectivities meet in clinical experience. The Freudian topics were more successful in representing the dynamics of individual psychic apparatuses. Inspired by aesthetic philosophy, Ferenczi imported the concept of empathy to describe a clinical style that considered a mixing zone between psyches. Winnicott, on the other hand, advanced in his attempt to describe the analytic space as a third area of experience, neither internal nor external, transitional. His reader Thomas Ogden invented the intersubjective analytic third to describe the *locus* of origin of the thoughts that emerge in the *setting*. Lucas Krüger is part of this tradition, using the conceptual metaphor of the "cloud state".

The conceptual metaphor is guided less by the ambition to create a new topology than by a tool to sensitise the reader and convey the author's understanding of the creative perspective of the psychoanalytic clinic. The "cloud state" is thus the condition of possibility for the analysand and analyst to be able to pass through intra- and intersubjective *customs*, making the psychoanalytic experience an event that effectively transforms ways of being, feeling and acting in the world.

The couch described by Krüger therefore has a richness that justifies it becoming the greatest symbol of Freudian invention. It is *Diwan*, both the writer and the poetic work: the place where the things that really matter are decided. It is the mother's body, the skin that forms the experience of madness. It allows the emergence of the child in the adult, regression and dreaming. It favours the ability to hate and survive hatred, anonymity and secrecy. It is the mirror that recognises our pain and our power. It is the protective hiding place – the boat, the castle – of children's play. It is the place where drive-related, representational and affective commerce is possible.

Surprisingly, Lucas Krüger publishes his book against the backdrop of the history of psychoanalysis, just when, after the COVID-19 pandemic, remote consultations became commonplace, mostly without the materiality of the couch – even though many analysands and analysts preferred the voice without an image, and others simulated couches in their private spaces.[2] However, considering the questions in *The Psychoanalytic Couch*, it is legitimate to ask whether, on the day when the couch is dispensable or no longer has a place in clinical listening spaces, there will still be something psychoanalytic in our culture.

Writing

I imagine our author on the couch in a "cloud state", fighting his critical ghosts and his fantasies of omnipotence, an enraged Quixote, relying on his Sancho Panza, also in a "cloud state", who listens to him and helps him confront and dispel his delusions, in order to find the right formula for them to become conceptual metaphors that are generous to the psychoanalytic community.

It was necessary for Lucas Krüger to divide his book into two distinct parts: Part I, "Listening perspectives", is dedicated to extensive and enviable academic research into the status of the couch in the work of various psychoanalysts. There are so many that I can't list them all here, but I can tell the reader that they will certainly find their favourite authors quoted. In Part II, "The poetics of psychoanalysis", Krüger seems to write as if his words were the fine rain that relieves us, announcing the end of the fury of a storm; it is the writing of someone who has certainly been in his theorising "cloud state" and has been able transmit, in an elaborate and stimulating way, what he has seen and intuited from there. We can see that Part I of the book, studious and obedient, gave Krüger the poetic licence to dare to think and write, from his theoretical-clinical *self*, the psychoanalysis he encountered on his journey with patients who inhabit the most diverse forms of suffering encountered by humans, from neurosis to narcissistic cleavages, from adults to children.

The psychoanalytic couch: Listening Perspectives and the Poetics of Psychoanalysis is therefore more than a book about the object that dominates the cultural imagination about what psychoanalysis is; it is a testament to the impact of psychoanalytic knowledge on someone who understands that this adventure is worth living, dreaming and passing on.

Daniel Kupermann is a psychoanalyst and professor in the department and graduate program of clinical psychology at the Institute of Psychology, University of São Paulo (USP). He is vice-president of the International Sándor Ferenczi Network, a founding member of the Brazilian Group for Sándor Ferenczi Studies and the author of several books on psychoanalysis.

Notes

1 According to the inspiration of the poetry of Murilo Mendes, quoted by Krüger, alongside many other poets who have dedicated themselves to the theme of the cloud.
2 Beyond the couch "proper", it should be emphasised that Krüger's proposal transcends the materiality of the couch and encompasses the experience of remote (online) analysis.

Opening

If there's one thing that represents psychoanalysis in popular culture and imagination, it's the couch. What is this couch really for? What is its function? These are laymen's questions ... but not only laymen. While its figure stands out, it also fuels the creation of dogmas and even taboos. It is therefore essential that we discuss in depth its specificities and its auxiliary functions in the psychoanalytic process.

It is a fact that Freud did little to theorise about the couch and its importance for listening and clinical intervention. There are rare and sparse moments in his work in which this object-furniture is mentioned, and the lack of theorisation about this important aid is, in fact, quite commonplace, even in the work of prominent authors.

Generally speaking, the authors don't bother to discuss the subject in depth, often devoting no more than a paragraph or two to the topic and, in the vast majority of cases, not even that. Therefore, due to the curious fact that to this day we still don't have a book that is fully committed to discussing the numerous and possible functions of the couch as an aid to analysis, this publication aims to fill this gap, with the purpose of presenting, by way of introduction, some *ways of listening and intervening from the couch*. And so, based on the exposition of different theoretical and clinical premises, we will ultimately identify unique perspectives on its functions. Although at many points we encounter antagonistic positions, we also find complementary ones that ultimately weave together layers of complexity, interconnecting them into a unified perspective on this object-furniture within psychoanalytic practice.

The notion of the frame, although fundamental to psychoanalytic theoretical and clinical thinking, is not the starting point of this discussion. Although this notion touches on the use of the couch – and, because of this, it will be present whenever necessary in the discussion – the purpose of this book is to delve into the specifics of the couch's functions. Writings that focus on the psychoanalytic frame, although extremely rich and important for thinking about psychoanalytic practice, usually "simplify" the couch as one of its constituent "elements",[1] and end up not developing some of the facets that we

DOI: 10.4324/9781003681212-1

intend to explore. This opening piece therefore sets out to shift the focus from the question of the frame to the couch itself, precisely in order to take account of specificities concerning the ways in which it is used in clinical practice, which end up not being properly contemplated when the focus is on the prism of the frame.

Thinking about the function of the couch is much more than thinking about elements of the frame, and this is what we intend to discuss throughout this book – although, obviously, the themes are interconnected. To this end, it is essential to take a historical look at how some possible functions of the couch were experienced and perceived by psychoanalysts in their work with their analysands, until they became part of their unique ways of listening and intervening throughout the development of psychoanalysis.

Compiling the contributions of some of the most important authors in psychoanalysis is essential if we are to understand the diversity and complexity of the ways of looking at the couch in the clinic, and this is one of the main objectives of the Part I of this book. In most cases, this task will require working with traces of embryonic ideas which, although present in written productions, are not the main topic of these texts. Guided by the sparse traces – which were not without their difficulties to piece together – we have mapped out some important contributions. If reflections on the use of the couch in the psychoanalytic session are already scarce in Sigmund Freud, they are no less so in Jacques Lacan, Wilfred Bion and Sándor Ferenczi, who devote only a sentence or two to the subject in their works. This is not very different from what we find in authors such as Donald Winnicott and Christopher Bollas, who, despite not devoting many paragraphs to the subject, make fundamental contributions that open new windows for us. We'll see how André Green, Thomas Ogden and René Roussillon start with reflections on the frame that culminate in a discussion of very important facets of working on the couch. We will also present Melanie Klein's efforts to understand and articulate the functions of the couch, even in the early days of psychoanalysis, without forgetting the contributions of Didier Anzieu, James Grotstein and John Munder Ross. In addition to the authors already mentioned, Chapter 14 comprises numerous contributions from authors such as Otto Rank, Karl Abraham, Otto Fenichel, Michael Balint, Donald Meltzer, Masud Khan, Jean Laplanche, César and Sara Botella, Antonino Ferro, Paula Heimann, Danielle Quinodoz and Hanna Segal, among many others.

Despite the aim of bringing together the contributions of all the authors mentioned, it must be emphasised that these chapters do not suffer from an opaque and aseptic neutrality on my part. Although it is of the utmost importance to be faithful to communicating the thinking of the selected authors as a whole, and it is my commitment to do so, their brief statements about the couch encourage us to listen beyond the gaps left and to follow the trails apparently not developed by them. Therefore, the book's aim transcends merely repeating the positions of others.

The psychoanalyst needs to listen "inside" psychoanalytic works in order to explore their gaps and penetrate their enigmas. From this perspective, I propose a "creative reading", as Thomas Ogden recommends,[2] in order to continue broadening the theoretical-clinical discussion. Consequently, alongside the presentation of these authors' contributions, points of reflection are raised which, in a way, weave threads that cross and interconnect the chapters, always with the aim of problematising the different perspectives on working with the couch and its functions, taking into account the singularities of each clinical case.

Part II, as well as complementing the discussions in Part I, brings angles of reflection not previously developed. If, on the one hand, it is constructed as a continuation of the previous discussion, on the other, it makes it clear that I undertook to work on the couch and its functions from what we could call "the poetics of psychoanalysis", which would culminate in discussing the poetic function contained in the work, from our auxiliary object-furniture. I must confess my difficulty in presenting the content of this second part in a brief introductory summary, as is the purpose of this "Opening", because I fear that listing the path to be followed will not help the reader's understanding much at the beginning, and could be seen as confusing.[3] However, this premise is also what makes it a bet, in terms of the psychoanalyst's work, because what is obscure in the clinic, especially in the first contacts with our analysands, is what drives us to remain curious and eager to continue our work. Curiosity is a powerful impetus for the psychoanalyst to keep listening to what may at first sound confusing, fragmentary and unfinished, and to follow the not-so-clear traces offered by the other, in order, perhaps, at some point, to reach some kind of clarification ... or perhaps not.

The starting point for these second ideas is to evoke the etymology of *diwan* (couch), which, curiously, was not developed by any of the authors researched and is apparently not known by other colleagues, despite the fact that it contains the essence of psychoanalytic practice. The Persian[4] aspect of *diwan* is closely linked to poetics and poetic work, while the Turkish-Ottoman aspect refers, among other meanings, to an "important meeting room" and to issues related to spatiality, as we will see later. Working from etymology will lead us to Goethe and his "cloud play", to rework different concepts linked to the functioning of the psyche, spatiality, poetics, the functions of play,[5] and to rearticulate notions involving *Verdichtung* (condensation), the *Dichter* (poet) and the *Dichtung* (poetic work), as well as construct a kind of *listening model* based on a metaphor that takes into account clouds, their movements and their morphology (among other aspects intrinsic to their figure). To this end, it would be no less important to work on the concept of *symbolic vesture*, which will help us to develop this clinical model of listening and intervention, closely related to the aspects discussed in Part I of the book, but also offering new perspectives of understanding to psychoanalytic work, based on the use of the couch.

Before proceeding with the chapters of this book, it is essential to caution the reader that all the discussion that follows ultimately gives precedence to the clinical work carried out in consulting rooms; nevertheless, it is by no means intended as an idealisation of the use of the couch.

The theme of the book has its limits and fails to encompass other modalities of psychoanalytic practice,[6] especially what is conventionally called "extramural psychoanalysis". I would like to emphasize the importance of psychoanalysis working in the social field and the creation of modalities that seek to work with psychoanalysis in different ways, be they, for example, group psychoanalysis or forms of work carried out in any environment other than the traditional clinic. I would like to express my deep respect for the seriousness of the colleagues dedicated to these modalities. With regard to this book, there are various accessibility issues that end up not being covered in depth, such as the lack of an in-depth discussion on listening to deaf analysands, who would need gestural-visual support in their communication. As for all these issues, I reiterate my conviction that there are colleagues better qualified to discuss them.

No less important than the previous caveat is the importance of recognising that, historically, psychoanalysis (and therefore treatment on the couch) has been more accessible to certain economic classes than to others. Fortunately, it seems to me that we are seeing more and more movements in favour of democratising access to treatment, especially with regard to financial (or even other) aspects.

Psychoanalysis is not and should not be a tool of power or exclusion. There is a lot to be done in this regard, and it is important to emphasise that rethinking the functions of the couch at a deep level is one way of not perpetuating dogmas about its use. In other words, the couch is an important auxiliary tool for listening; studying its functions in depth is also one of the ways of expanding access to treatments that make use of it.

At this point, it is necessary to contextualize that the use of the couch presupposes, first of all, a psychoanalyst. And a psychoanalyst is someone who has gone through or is going through[7] the basic process of the "analytical triad", which consists of in-depth theoretical study, supervision and a "good enough" analysis, if we can put that way. A psychoanalyst will always be formed from the relationship with the other, in a process that we could call "inside out" and not "outside in". As you can see, my way of presenting the issue is generic, as it is intended to cover the different models of training in psychoanalysis. I am talking about any and all consistent training in psychoanalysis, regardless of whether it is carried out using models linked to the IPA or Lacanian models, or whether it is carried out in other independent institutions[8] that are serious and committed to psychoanalytic practice. More than any institutional link, since there are also psychoanalysts who choose a path not connected to them – by dedicating themselves to the essential analytical triad – I'm referring to the fact that a psychoanalyst is always made from the "inside out" and through intense dedication. A psychoanalyst's training is never complete, but rather an uninterrupted process that accompanies them until the end of their journey.

Although the aim of this book isn't to discuss the details of psychoanalytic training, I can't ignore the fact that, unfortunately, we have witnessed the emergence of various false training courses, some of which are even bizarre, such as those called "evangelical psychoanalysis", or other types in which we don't find any psychoanalysis at all. Also worrying is the creation of "flash courses", which promise to train psychoanalysts in a few months, distorting the ethics and seriousness of psychoanalysis, without taking into account the fundamental analytical triad and deluding the unwary with superficial propaganda. We need to be vigilant and remember that, just as we cannot sacralise psychoanalysis, neither can we allow a serious and ethical practice to be trivialised.

I'll end this section by inviting the reader to browse through the reflections that permeate the following chapters, reiterating that this is an introductory study and will likely call for further dialogue among peers. Above all, I hope that this writing raises questions and awakens the desire of colleagues to keep problematising and discussing the couch.

Notes

1 As we'll see later, especially in Chapter 5, "André Green's couch: The dream model, other contributions and misreadings", the theme of the frame encompasses many elements, of which the couch is just one.
2 Ogden, 2014.
3 "I'm explaining to you to confuse you / I'm confusing you to enlighten you", sings Tom Zé in the chorus of his song *Tô*, from the album *Estudando o samba* (1976).
4 Mario Coutinho Jorge and Antonio Quinet briefly mention Persian ethnology in their books, although they don't develop it, or at least not in the way I propose (see Jorge, 2017; Quinet, 2009).
5 I am referring here to play in its broadest sense, taking into account Freud's use of the word *Spiel*, as explained by the translator Paulo César de Sousa. "The word *Spiel*, which corresponds to the English word *play*, can be translated as 'play', 'game', 'musical performance' or 'theatrical representation'" [Freud, (1942, (1905/1906)) 2019a, p. 363]. Portuguese lacks a single term with the semantic breadth of *Spiel* or *play*, and the present passage seeks to elucidate this.
6 Including remote (online) counselling, which is better covered in the discussion in the second part of the book and, above all, in the extra chapter in the endmatter, "Provocative considerations on remote online sessions: The need for the couch or a substitute other than the gaze".
7 I'm talking about colleagues who are still in the initial process of psychoanalytic training, but are practising as analysts with their own analysands.
8 As is the case with me.

PART I

Listening perspectives

Chapter 1

Sigmund Freud's couch-reminiscence

We can't discuss the couch in psychoanalysis without first reflecting on Freud's use of this instrument. Although the couch became essential in his psychoanalytic practice and has naturally been incorporated by all psychoanalysts since then, Freud's writings mention it rarely. The best ideas don't always come about in an elaborate way, and the use of the couch corroborates this statement, since it wasn't a resource initially thought up for psychoanalytic practice, but rather a "remnant of the hypnotic method",[1] as Freud prefers to summarise it. In fact, his couch was given to him as a gift by a patient (Madame Benvenisti) at the beginning of the 1890s, according to historian and biographer Peter Gay, based on comments made by Marie Bonaparte – even before the word *psychoanalysis* appeared for the first time in 1896, in *The Heredity and Aetiology of Neuroses*. According to Gay,[2] Freud's couch was itself a "spectacle":[3]

> The glass shelves were full of books and covered with objects; the walls were lined with snapshots and daguerreotypes. The famous couch was a spectacle in itself, piled high with cushions, with a rug at the foot for patients to use if they felt cold, and covered with a Persian rug, a Shiraz.[4]

However, beyond the facts and Freud's description of the couch, let's also try to read/listen to the complexity of his apparently simple statement that the couch is a "remnant of the hypnotic method". The idea of the couch being a remnant, therefore a reminiscence of another period, makes perfect sense if we think about the way Freud viewed the clinic, doesn't it? Throughout this chapter, I invite the reader to discuss a few questions, including the one initially raised.

Firstly, let's point out that the founder of psychoanalysis will accompany us throughout the rest of the chapters and authors in this first part, as well as the ideas proposed in the second part. This makes this chapter just an initial provocation for discussion. Little by little, as the book goes on, we will re-discuss and reveal other functions of the couch that can be "found" within Freudian theory. To this end, I ask the reader to be patient and to stay with the first

DOI: 10.4324/9781003681212-3

questions raised in this chapter, waiting for them to become more complex by the end of our journey.

The status of the couch lies in an unwritten gap in Freud's work, and only allows us to imagine what might be present in this "blank space", since Freud never discussed it from the point of view of metapsychology. Let's start by recalling his words in *Recommendations to Physicians Practising Psycho-Analysis*:[5]

> However, I must make it clear that what I am saying is that this technique is the only one appropriate to my individuality; I don't risk denying that a doctor who is constituted in an entirely different way might be led to adopt a different attitude towards his patients and the task at hand.

Freud developed a technical way of working that was appropriate for him as an analyst, but not necessarily for other analysts. In this way, he shows that the uniqueness of the analyst is fundamental to the use of technical resources and indicates that it is possible for another psychoanalyst to find different ways of carrying out an analysis, not necessarily the same ones that he, Freud, found. The development of child analysis and a whole new range of resources and listening possibilities that have opened up as a result serve as excellent examples of these different ways of working psychoanalytically.

On Beginning the Treatment[6] is the only text in which Freud reflects on the use of the couch. Right at the start, he warns us that his recommendations should not be followed unconditionally. It is in his interest that there should be reflection on them, critical and clinical thinking on the part of the reader-analyst in order to justify his practices. It is in this text that the founder of psychoanalysis shares with his readers that the couch is not a resource initially designed for analytical practice, but rather a remnant of the hypnotic method. Although it may seem simple, Freud's seemingly naïve remark is curious, as it carries the idea of an object that contains a trace of another moment, of another mode of functioning.

As if talking to the reader "freely", Freud is demonstrating what the couch means to him as an analyst: an object that contains a trace of another moment/time/functioning. The fact that the couch-object refers to a previous trace cannot be seen as insignificant.

I believe that to think about the couch in Freud is, first and foremost, to think of it through the prism of reminiscences. That is why I propose that we reflect on its use as being intrinsically linked to what each analyst considers to be the object – and the objective – of analysis.[7] Emphasising the remnant character of the couch makes perfect sense if we think about Freud's clinical legacy. Even with some theoretical reconfigurations made over time, it's possible to say that his fundamental clinical thinking turns on the idea of something from the past that is living in the present. In fact, this formula (of the past persisting in the present) is a way of trying to explain the inexplicable (no matter how hard we try) and only experiential *transference*.[8] There is a trace that remains and lives in the present, even when imperceptible.

If, as we are thinking, the couch has its own historical reminiscences, when we reflect on Freud's clinical practice, we will conclude that he listened to a person with their traces, lying on an instrument-object-furniture with their traces. Could we be looking at a couch-vehicle for travelling through history, for travelling back in time, a vehicle of affection, a trace that links the Unconscious to the transference? We could infer that the couch is the "ideal" piece of furniture and work object for Freud, due to its transferential meaning of "past trace", but he never wrote this down. It's just an attempt to listen to something latent from an imaginative listening that tries to grasp what lies beyond the manifest. It seems fundamental to a psychoanalyst to place imagining as an important function in the creation of hypotheses in the work of analysis. This question of imagination will be looked at more closely once we've moved on to other contributions. André Green, by the way, provides an excellent interpretation, from another angle, of the function of the couch, based on the dream model of Freudian metapsychology.[9]

Let's not forget the central role of sexuality in Freudian theory; and just as we have suggested Freud's use of the couch because of its historical traces, we could easily suggest its use due to sexuality. The couch alludes to the bed – an intimate place where sexual relations commonly take place, and its horizontality refers to the sexual relationship itself. This is also a fundamental facet for working on the transferential relationship. Consequently, the couch would facilitate the emergence of infantile sexuality and genitality, which, in fact, is a central issue in hysteria, a pathology to which Freud devoted a great deal of attention. The bed has been an intimate place since childhood – even from birth – and its connection with infantile sexuality and partial drives would also be contemplated and facilitated through the use of the couch.

In other words, we could say that the couch is the vehicle for the return of the repressed. Lying on it, the analysand would manifest – via displacement and condensation and by making use of the transference to the analyst – latent contents of his or her primal experiences, of his or her infantile sexuality. It is from these manifest contents in session that the analytical process would take place, since it is the manifest contents, disguised by the action of repression, that have allowed for the access to psychoanalytic work involving unconscious contents. In other words, the use of the couch would be consonant with the clinic of neurotic pathologies.

Returning to *On Beginning the Treatment*, we note that Freud shared that he couldn't bear to be stared at for many hours. When listening to an analysand, he would surrender himself to "the current of his own unconscious thoughts" and would not wish his facial expressions to influence the analysand's free association. For him, this could be felt as a nuisance by the analysand, especially if a scopic impulse plays an important role in their neurosis. Freud stated that he was aware many analysts worked without the piece of furniture, but he could not confirm whether they did so out of a desire to act differently or because, in some way, it seemed advantageous for them to do so. Even though many analysands resisted the use of the couch – generally because they did not want to stop seeing the analyst – Freud preferred to refuse face-to-face treatment.[10] He insisted on the use of the couch because of the transference, since it has "the purpose and the result of preventing the inadvertent intrusion of the transference into the patient's spontaneous thoughts, of isolating the transference and making it stand out clearly as resistance in due course".[11] From this perspective, we are also led to think of the couch as a kind of protector of the "neutrality" defended by Freud, trying to demarcate a separation between what is of one psyche and what is of another in the processes of analysis.

Despite imaginative efforts to find latent meanings for Freud's use of the couch – supported by his theory but not explicitly stated by him – we cannot deny that it is, in fact, his personal motivations and limitations (his discomfort with the gaze), and not metapsychological motives, that he shares as his justification for its use. Such an observation helps us to think about not neglecting the analyst's discomforts and difficulties. The discomfort with the analysand's gaze, as reported by Freud, indicates that the analyst's quality of listening may be impaired by this gaze of the other, which would act as yet another element to be processed by the analyst – that is, an excess.

The couch is intended to safeguard the quality of listening – of floating attention – and also to protect the analysand's free association.[12] Using the couch would be a way of taking due care that the analyst's possible reactions don't disturb the analysand's free association and negatively influence the treatment. From this perspective, therefore, the couch would be an artifice so that the analyst doesn't get in the way of the analysand's process.

Beyond these considerations, we must keep raising the question: Why use the couch, and to what end? Let us keep reflecting on these initial provocations, in light of the contributions that follow.

Notes

1 Freud, (1913a) 1996e, p. 149.
2 Gay, 1989, p. 168.
3 An understanding of the order of this "spectacle" would be linked to the staging of a "play" of the Unconscious, which will be further developed in Part II of this book.
4 A discussion about the functionality of inanimate objects in the analyst's room as aids to the analytical process is developed by Christopher Bollas, as will be seen in Part I, Chapter 7, "Christopher Bollas and the evocative couch". The use of blankets or similar to cover oneself during the analysis session is commented on by Winnicott and Didier Anzieu, as we will see in the chapters that aim to bring their contributions to the table (Part I, Chapter 3, "The couch-body of Donald Woods Winnicott" and Part I, Chapter 4, "Didier Anzieu's skin couch"), but is also found in other authors, who will be mentioned later. In *Recommendations to Physicians*

Practising Psychoanalysis, there is a passage in which Freud points out that the analysand occupies himself mentally with the "appearance of the room", "thinks about the objects in the consulting room" and the fact that he is lying on the couch [Freud, (1912) 1996d, p. 153].

5 Freud, (1912) 1996d, p. 125.

6 Freud, (1913a) 1996e, p. 139.

7 This proposition should become clearer when the thoughts of other psychoanalysts are presented in subsequent parts of this book.

8 Although, as we should know, working via the transferential field also includes working with the "new", which comes from the unique encounter between the analysand and the analysed.

9 André Green's proposal is based on Freud's metapsychology, but it should be seen as Green's original contribution, since Freud did not establish the very interesting correlations between the use of the couch and his metapsychology, as Green has done. We'll look at André Green's conjectures in Part I, Chapter 5, "André Green's couch: The dream model, other contributions and misreadings", remembering that not only Green deals with thinking about the function of the couch, taking Freud as his starting point.

10 Freud, (1913a) 2010, p. 186.

11 Freud, (1913b) 2010, p. 179.

12 This issue is further developed in Part I, Chapter 6, "Thomas Ogden and privacy on the couch".

Chapter 2

The couch, the child who lives in the adult, and the technical daring of Sándor Ferenczi

If discussing the use of the couch was not frequent in Freud's extensive body of work, it was even less so in the work of his contemporaries. Ferenczi, always daring in his experimentation with the psychoanalytic technique, brings up some passages that can open up ways of thinking about its use (or non-use). Although the couch accompanied his entire clinical practice, and Ferenczi never questioned its importance, we will see how he sometimes "deviated" from its use. I've compiled his sparse notes so that we can problematise them, in order to try to find the essence of his thinking about the function of the couch and analysis as a whole.

In *Principle of Relaxation and Neocatharsis*,[1] Ferenczi calls himself, although it's not true, a "transgressor"[2] of Freud's "technical advice". One of the reasons for this "transgression" would be to occasionally allow an analysand to get up, wander around his room and leave the couch when they felt the need to say something while looking into Ferenczi's eyes.

This consideration, among others that will be addressed, can be regarded as a motivation for some analysts to advocate face-to-face treatment rather than the couch, especially in the clinical cases that Ferenczi would call "difficult cases". However, I believe the matter can be understood in a broader and less simplistic way, and we will need to go through to the end of the chapter to reach such an understanding.

"Wandering" through the space of the consulting room seems to be totally in keeping with child analysis, which was structuring its foundations as a modality of care,[3] making the necessary technical changes in relation to the "classic" way of looking at analysis. The acceptance that the analysand occupies the *room/setting* in its entirety, explores it, wanders through it, and uses it extensively is essential in the children's clinic. This was something that Ferenczi, Melanie Klein's first analyst (one of the forerunners of this modality), did not neglect in his listening to adults.

If you'll allow me to adopt a more conversational tone, since we're among colleagues, I think it's interesting to point out that when I first read Ferenczi's phrase about "wandering" in the space of analysis, it touched me deeply. Since

DOI: 10.4324/9781003681212-4

the beginning of my clinical practice, I have treated both adults and children. As you know, children make more use of the consulting room than adults do – from a physical point of view, at least. Therefore, from the outset, because I thought of the freedom with which child analysands naturally took up the space of analysis to express themselves, I had an imaginative thought of a trapeze artist in analysis, lying upside down on a trapeze[4] (instead of lying on the couch).

In the children's clinic, many auxiliary toy objects are offered during the session. The question arose as to why an adult couldn't use the session in creatively[5] similar ways – like being upside down, for example. This playful reverie served – and still serves – as a stimulus for many questions: What is an analysis? What is no longer an analysis? What is an analysis for? How can an analysis be made? How can an analysis not be made? These are questions that incite us to think about our practice and our work ethic.

We could reflect for hours on this trapeze imaginative thought, even from a foetal point of view, as if we are all "floating" in the womb and even upside down – at least at the moment of birth.[6] All daydreams have the potential to lead us to new ideas, but not all of them can or should necessarily come true. So, for me, the respective daydream fulfils more of a metaphorical function than anything else, and since I've never seen a trapeze artist, the daydream has never been more than a stimulus for reflecting on analytical practice and the aids to analysis that we have at our disposal in our consulting rooms.

In *Preliminaries to the active technique*,[7] Ferenczi presents a clinical case in which singing and playing the piano in a session helped to unveil aspects of the analysand's sexuality and childhood conflicts, closely linked to her body and her bodily activity, which involved controlling her anal and urethral sphincters, as well as clitoral masturbation. We wouldn't be interested in discussing Ferenczi's active technique here,[8] nor would we want to go into the details of the case. However, it is interesting to think about what is implied: the musical instrument used as an extension of the body. When describing how man built civilisation and his tools, Freud[9] states that "through each instrument, man recreates his own organs, motor or sensory, or extends the limits of their functioning". Although Freud isn't referring to the musical instrument itself, the statement certainly includes it.[10] So we have to ask ourselves: Couldn't we think of the couch, an instrument (in the broad sense) of the psychoanalyst, from the corporeal perspective alluded to by Freud?

In *Technical Difficulties of an Analysis of Hysteria*,[11] Ferenczi tells us of a case in which an analysand would covertly masturbate by rubbing her legs during the treatment (on the couch). Given that it was a case of hysteria, couldn't she be taking the couch as an analogue of the bed (where sexual relations take place) or even as a substitute object for the father's and/or analyst's body? I'll let these questions reverberate in the reader's mind, in order to revisit them later in light of Winnicott's conception of the couch, as we'll see in the next chapter.

There are also other fragments of Ferenczi's work that help us to problematise the use of the couch. In one of these passages, he writes about lengthening sessions and/or having more than one session a day with some analysands, due, among other reasons, to the "shock effect of the brutal interruption of the analysis session",[12] explaining that it is possible, when a session is over, for the analysand, "comfortably settled in with your analyst",[13] to be wrenched out of a dream and strongly affected by the experience, to the point of even showing symptoms as a result. Ferenczi had a keen ear for the effects of the analytical process and for how lying on the couch could lead to feeling as though one was inside a dream, while the end of the session and the consequent departure from the couch would tear the analysand out of this "materialised dream".

The idea that the session and its devices assist in entering the dream world is also present in *The Analysis of Adults with Children*[14] – a text derived from an extraordinary lecture at the Vienna Psychoanalytic Society on the occasion of Freud's 75th birthday. There, Ferenczi writes: "we even let the patient immerse himself in all the early stages of passive object love, where, in murmured phrases, like a child about to fall asleep, he allows us to glimpse his oneiric universe."[15] However, in addition to entering a oneiric world, Ferenczi is elucidating the function of the couch as a way of accessing and regressing to "early stages of passive object love". This can be understood as a regression to a stage of initial fusion between the baby and its mother; a state of bodily and psychic undifferentiation; a primitive stage of being and/or a stage of vulnerability, revealing the important function of the couch for accessing and re-elaborating primitive experiences or moments of traumatic vulnerability.[16]

When Ferenczi sets out to attend to the child who lives in the adult, he proposes an *analysis through play*.[17] He tells us, for example, of a case in which, during a session, an analysand hugs him and, whispering and narrating a scene, calls him Grandpa – prompting Ferenczi to play the role of Grandpa (evoked by the analysand), continuing the scene, whispering too.[18] In fact, based on his reports, some of his analyses could involve touch, role-playing and – as he himself points out during the conference at the Vienna Psychoanalytic Society – drawings made by the analysands, without him believing that he was violating psychoanalytic ethics. These dramatisations of childhood experiences (performances at the level of unburdening, in some cases) and/or the *primitive drawings* offered by the analysands to Ferenczi would be – if we summarise his thinking as much as possible – a way of reliving the trauma (accompanied by the analyst), to work through it, and to reconcile divided parts of the psyche. Accepting the analysand's demand, however primitive and narcissistic it may be, is part of the analyst's role, regardless of the auxiliary devices available in the session.

As can be noted, instead of following a continuous line of thought on the couch, it is necessary to listen/read between the lines of Ferenczi's work to find clues and fragments of considerations on its use or non-use. However, they are fragments that contain embryos for our reflection, especially if we think that, even today, only a few analysts take the time to reflect and write more deeply on the subject.

Ferenczi was a great experimenter and spared no effort in trying to develop psychoanalytic theory and practice; however, despite his successes, we also find failures. To give in to a so-called "preference" and the desire of the analysand can also become the practice of non-analysis. We see this reach its ultimate consequences when, towards the end of his life, Ferenczi started working on the basis of a mutual analysis between analyst and analysand – something initially desired and proposed by an analysand – which turned out to be a disastrous experience.

His lesson leaves us with questions such as: Is the analysand's preference (manifest desire) something that must be followed by the analyst in analysis? Bringing this question to the contemporary dichotomy of couch *versus* face-to-face: Is giving up the couch in favour of face-to-face or another modality a question that depends on the "preference" of the analysand and their manifest desire? If the analysand claims to "prefer" to see the analyst, would that be a reason to carry out a face-to-face treatment? Or is this "preference" at the service of their symptomatology, even if it turns out to be serious, and we need to think about it from another angle? Should we listen to their words or what's behind them?

Even though Ferenczi[19] claims eventually to allow the analysand to leave the couch to say something while looking into his, Ferenczi's, eyes, and there are other reports of clinical situations outside the couch – such as the aforementioned piano playing and role-playing combined with playing ("analysis through play") – it would be untrue to say that he sought to contemplate an the use of face-to-face to the detriment of the couch. We won't find any theoretical position on his part that supports a defence of the importance of the concrete gaze. It's remarkable how his psychoanalytic work takes place *primarily* on the couch. I understand that his "elasticity of technique"[20] is much more related to the idea of facilitating the emergence of the child who lives in the adult than to any reflection on the importance of the concrete gaze (because the analyst "looks" when listening, and the analysand is "looked at" when listened to),[21] although it is also untrue to say that Ferenczi was opposed to consultations, since his work is characterised by experimentation.

I understand that the essence of his thinking is to emphasise the importance of play as an aid to the analysis of adults too, and this would not necessarily involve a proposal to defend a modality head on. For Ferenczi, it is important for the analysand to feel at ease to be as they are, without feeling subjected to the other. If the couch were to take the place of an object of power for the analyst, Ferenczi would certainly give it up, since his fight was always against totalitarianism and abuses of power, which shows that the use of the couch should never serve these purposes. We do know, however, that Ferenczi dedicated himself to welcoming and listening to a wide variety of clinicians on the couch, without at any time theorising any problem with its use.

Therefore, even though examples have been pointed out outside a more "classical" context, it is important to emphasise that Ferenczi's work does not advocate alternative devices that undermine the use of the couch. He proposes the acceptance and expansion of new possibilities (if the couch comes to occupy a role of power, of submission of the analysand to the analyst, and puts the analysand at the mercy of possible cold treatment by the analyst). He proposes that the analyst should welcome the child that lives in the adult, so the use (or not) of the couch should also take this aspect into account.[22]

Notes

1 Ferenczi, (1930) 1992a.
2 Ferenczi, (1930) 1992a, p. 58.
3 Although Hermine von Hugh-Hellmuth became the first psychoanalyst for children in 1908, and it is possible to think of Freud's work with Little Hans in 1905 as a precursor of the practice, it was from the 1920s onwards that the modality was better developed through the contributions of Melanie Klein and Anna Freud.
4 Leopoldo Nosek humorously quotes an analysand of his who "defended" the idea of conducting his analysis *online* while on his skateboard. [Nosek said this at the launch event for the book by Anna Staal and Howard Levine, *Psicanálise e vida covidiana: desamparo coletivo, experiência individual* (Blucher, 2021), broadcast via YouTube on 2 June 2021.]
5 There are very important functions in using the couch from a creative point of view, and we'll see this throughout the book, especially in Part II.
6 Here, I'm referring to ideal conditions, relating them to the metaphor of the trapeze artist. Of course, there are various complications surrounding a birth, and there are many cases when the baby is not in the healthy position expected for labour.
7 Ferenczi, (1921) 2011a, pp. 117–135.
8 For a more in-depth understanding of Sándor Ferenczi's work, I would recommend reading Daniel Kupermann's publications, in particular the books *Why Ferenczi?* (2019) and *Sensitive Presence: Care and Creation in the Psychoanalytic Clinic* (2021), among other publications in journals.
9 Freud, (1930) 2006a, p. 97.
10 In *Clinical Sonorities* (Krüger, 2017), I tried to elucidate, based on various clinical situations, some specific functions that particular musical instruments can fulfil in analyses with children, especially in questions related to the body (Krüger, 2017).
11 Ferenczi, (1919) 2011.
12 Ferenczi, (1930) 1992a, p. 58.
13 Ferenczi, (1915) 2019, p. 57.
14 Ferenczi, (1931) 2011b, p. 69.
15 Ferenczi, (1931) 2011b, p. 78.
16 A facet explored by Winnicott, as we'll see below.
17 Ferenczi, (1931) 2011b, p. 69.
18 This specific situation will be taken up again in Part II, when we articulate, among other issues, what *Darstellung* and symbolic vesture are all about.
19 Ferenczi, (1930) 1992a, p. 58.
20 Ferenczi, (1928) 1992.
21 Nasio makes a similar comment: "Seeing is not looking, but I would also say: vision must be excluded from the space of the analytic session so that the gaze has greater power, so that the gaze is a strong and powerful gaze" (Nasio, 1995, p. 15).
22 The proposal to work with the child who lives in the adult is central to Part II of this book.

Chapter 3

The couch-body of Donald Woods Winnicott

Although he didn't write specifically on the subject, Winnicott's contribution in relation to the couch is fruitful. Let's start with the texts "Hate in Countertransference" (1947) and "Metapsychological and Clinical Aspects of Regression within the Psycho-Analytical Set-Up" (1954a), in which he makes important points. I'll comment after transcribing the significant passages:

> The couch and cushions are there for the patient to use. They will appear in thoughts and dreams, and in this case they will represent the analyst's body, their breasts, arms, hands, etc. in an infinite variety of forms. To the extent that the patient is regressed (for a moment or an hour, or over a long period of time) the couch is the analyst, the pillows *are* breasts, the analyst *is* the mother at a certain time in the past. In extreme situations, the couch can no longer be said to represent the analyst.[1]
>
> For the neurotic, the couch, warmth and comfort can *symbolise* the mother's love. For the psychotic, it would be more accurate to say that these things are the physical expression of the analyst's love. The couch is the analyst's lap or womb, and the warmth is the warmth of the analyst's body – and so on.[2]

In these passages, Winnicott makes it clear that the couch can be seen from two different, paradoxical, yet complementary angles essential for a complete understanding. For example, the couch can be performing the function of *representing* a mother object, just as it can be perceived as *being* the mother – in other words, he places it in a paradox of "being" and "representing". His proposition includes the use of the couch within a spectrum of the greatest depth and even combining it with a primitivity that the psyche of the analysand can achieve in a sufficiently well-conducted analysis.

Beyond a more "classical" use, Winnicott conceives the couch as a body. This couch-body can come to occupy the transferential role that the analyst would occupy: the body of the analyst/mother – a body that supports fragile primitiveness.

DOI: 10.4324/9781003681212-5

Winnicott's theoretical thinking is always characterised by paradox – there are coexistences. And it is in this way that the couch can, at the same time, be taken by the analysand as furniture, but also as the body of the mother, or even as the body of the mother-analyst, if we think of the transference. In these passages, Winnicott refers to the analysand as the primary object (maternal function), but this leaves us open to ask ourselves, when it comes to the role of the analyst in the transference, whether it wouldn't also be possible to think about this status of the body from the perspective of genital sexuality and neurotic conflict. As we saw in the previous chapter, Ferenczi deals with a case in which an analysand masturbated in disguise by rubbing her legs against each other during the consultation, while lying on the couch. I reiterate the question from the previous chapter: wouldn't the analysand, described as hysterical, be taking the couch as a substitute for the body of the father and/or the analyst? Let's continue, letting the question reverberate. Returning directly to Winnicott's statements, note the italics he uses: depending on the case and the situation, the couch can *represent a body*, while in other cases it *would be perceived as a body*. In other words, in the passages quoted, Winnicott is presenting us with two ways of relating to the object-couch. In one of them, the analysand takes the couch as a representation of the mother's and/or analyst's body. In the other, the analysand takes the couch to be the body of the mother and/or the analyst, and each form depends on the psyche of the analysand and their regression in analysis. We are talking about a couch-object-body that *represents holding* or that *does/is holding*, depending on the analysand's need for and use of the instrument-couch. From the perspective of the primary object, the couch is – it personifies – the body that supports the analysand during regression.

When on the couch, the analysand is supported by a "body". So perhaps we could say that it is through this "body" – the couch and cushions – and its cosiness that the analysand gives themself up to analysis and regression. It's a paradox because, on the one hand, the analysand is lying "alone", but on the other hand, they are supported bodily. From this paradoxical perspective, the couch *is* and *is not* the body of the mother/analyst and can also fulfil, from Winnicott's theoretical perspective, a function as a transitional object – as well as being, radically, the skin that covers it[3] or even the womb/capsule that contains it.

Margarett Little[4] reports that, in her analysis with Winnicott, she was on the couch at times of extreme regression, completely covered by a blanket, holding hands with the analyst.

> Literally, for endless hours, he held my two hands tightly between his, almost like an umbilical cord, while I lay there, often hidden under the blanket, silent, inert, withdrawn, terrified, angry or in tears, sleeping and sometimes dreaming.[5]

"For me, D.W. didn't represent my mother. In my illusion of transference, he was my mother. As there is in fact continuity between mother and foetus, genetic and physical, for me his hands were the umbilical cord; his couch was the placenta; and the blanket, the membranes ....”[6] This and other accounts by Little resonate with Winnicott’s comments about the couch, reinforcing that, in his view, the couch is an auxiliary instrument to analysis in any kind of psychic suffering. The couch is there to be used in whatever way the analysand needs, symbolically or not, bodily or not, neurotically or not. The accounts of Margaret Little’s analysis lead us to understand the couch as the body of the other that helps the *self* and/or the psyche to develop.

Today we know,[7] due to advances in medicine, that the tactile and auditory senses are prominent in the life of the foetus, and that it even dreams of “sound images”. The rhythm of the mother’s and foetus’ heartbeats, as well as the blood flow, are present from the tactile bodily vibration of intrauterine life and become more complex as the auditory system develops. Winnicott probably already intuited the importance of this tactile-auditory primitiveness, opening up the possibility of thinking of the use of the couch (and listening from it) as an instrument-object of support, an instrument that can be complementary to and/or an extension of the body, just like in the mother-baby relationship.

It’s important to emphasise that in her book, Little reports intense suffering, and she calls herself a borderline psychotherapist. In her previous analyses, being on the couch was experienced as a terrifying experience – which was not the case in her treatment on Winnicott’s couch. This issue is extremely important for the discussion of the contemporary dichotomy about the indication of the couch *versus* face-to-face treatments in non-neurotic cases. From Winnicott’s perspective, the “problem” would not be whether or not to use the couch in serious cases, but rather how the analyst would listen and intervene in these cases, even on the couch. Otherwise, how could we explain the fact that in one analysis the use of the couch would evoke the terrifying, but in another it would fulfil the role that Little reports in her analysis with Winnicott?

We could think, with the help of Ferenczi’s *Einfühlung*, that we need to be connected to the other person’s suffering in order to listen to them. As Winnicott points out, the couch is not an obstacle if the intervention is in line with the way the analysand needs to be listened to. Certainly, we are talking about a *setting* that embraces the potential for play, just as in analysing children, in which the objects in the consulting room can acquire properties beyond their original ones.

Winnicott’s theory and listening are intrinsically connected. In *Retreat and Regression*,[8] we can see how he describes clinical situations that emphasise the corporeal-object issue of the couch. In this text, there is a description of an analysand who rolls and shrinks on the couch *like a foetus inside his mother’s womb*, according to the author’s conception. His interpretation (supported by other clinical data) was that the analysand, as well as regressing to *his original dependence on his mother*, was identifying at that moment with his own child, which was developing inside his wife.

At a later point in the same analysis, he goes on to say that, for the analysand, "the couch had automatically become the analyst's lap".[9] Since the aim is not to destroy this analysis, but only to elucidate the status of the couch in Winnicott's thinking, let's point out how, in this case too, the couch plays a *holding* role and presents itself as an object available to be used as the psyche of the analysand needs it – or, in other words, as the *self* needs it to develop.

Winnicott explains that regression to dependence is "an integral part of the analysis of early childhood phenomena, and if the couch gets wet, the patient gets dirty or drools, we will know that these things are inherent, not a complication".[10] His thinking demonstrates the breadth of his listening and the extent of his psychic availability to what comes from the analysand.

There are contemporary psychoanalysts who rely on Winnicott's theorizations to affirm the need for some treatments to be face-to-face, although he never brought the subject up for discussion in these terms. It's important to emphasise that this movement is more about how some may interpret Winnicott's work than, in fact, his recommendations; after all, according to the excerpts here, we see Winnicott using the couch with adult patients, finding a function for the couch within his theoretical-clinical context. Just the fact that he sees children, sees patients in hospital and does therapeutic consultations[11] already signals to us that the couch is not his only tool. Of course, he doesn't affirm the couch as a unique tool to detriment of others, but neither does he advocate not using it. Winnicott is concerned with signalling that there is no "problem" in the patient regressing on the couch, on the contrary, the "problem" would be the analyst's unpreparedness for such a situation.

> It is commonly thought that a patient's regression in analysis poses some danger. The danger is not in the regression but in the analyst's unpreparedness to deal with the regression and the dependency that is part of it. When an analyst has had an experience that makes him confident in his handling of regression, then it can probably be said that the more quickly the analyst accepts regression and makes full contact with it, the less likely the patient will need to penetrate an illness with regressive qualities.[12]

In *Aims of Psychoanalytic Treatment*,[13] Winnicott claims to carry out a *modified analysis*.[14] Even without directly specifying what this would mean, he reiterates that, although he tries to follow a *standard analysis* as much as possible,[15] he is not afraid to "practise something else"[16] if necessary.

> I find myself working as an analyst rather than carrying out standard analysis when I'm faced with certain conditions that I've learned to recognise:

a) When the fear of madness dominates the picture.
b) When a false *self* becomes successful, and the façade of success, however shiny, has to be demolished at some stage for the analysis to be successful.

c) When, in a patient, an antisocial tendency, whether in the form of aggression, theft or both, is the legacy of deprivation.
d) When there is no cultural life, only a reality and a relationship with external reality, the two being relatively disconnected.
e) When a sick father or mother dominates the picture.[17]

Winnicott leaves it unclear what this *modified analysis* would be for *special cases*. This may give readers the opportunity to interpret that the opposite of his statement about *standard analysis* is analysis without a couch. However, the careful reader of Winnicott's text will easily realise that, when he refers to *standard analysis*, he is referring to the use of the technique of interpretation as a resource for the analyst. He questions the effectiveness of interpretation – in the Freudian sense, a technique for bringing out the latent (unconscious) meaning of session material with the aim of bringing it to the consciousness of the analysand through verbal/oral communication from the analyst.[18]

In other words, what Winnicott sets out to discuss as *modified analysis* is not the status of the couch as a tool, but rather the analyst's handling of clinical situations. Winnicott is talking about transcending interpretation as a technique; it is management and not the use or non-use of the couch that is the essence of the discussion he proposes, and he would add: "I modify myself in the sense of being a psychoanalyst who satisfies, or tries to satisfy, the needs of a special case. I believe that this non-analytic work can best be done by an analyst who is versed in classical psychoanalytic technique."[19] An important statement, but I would disagree with the term "non-analytic work"; after all, Winnicott's technique is in favour of the deepest psychoanalysis. What Winnicott proposes are broad ways of dealing with the *setting* and its auxiliary objects. In this way, he considered the use of the couch in its non-verbal facet, expanding its use beyond the classic form, which prioritises the word as an intervention. For him, it's not necessarily a question of giving up the couch when treating more difficult cases – although he has no qualms about this – it's a question of seeing other potential uses for the couch beyond the classic model – to listen and intervene in other ways. His clinical practice shows us that each theoretical conception and intervention is closely linked to a unique way of listening.

Therefore, in addition to its classic use, Winnicott's contribution to the subject allows us to think about the potential of the couch for non-neurotic cases as well, avoiding a simplifying equation of neurosis/couch *versus* non-neurosis/couch. **It is the analyst's way of listening to the analysand on the couch that determines how it is used**, showing that it is not question of problematising the issue of severe cases solely on the basis of a simplistic idea of whether or not to use this object-furniture.

It's interesting that not even in the text *The mirror role of the mother and the family in child development*,[20] full of clinical cases, which deals with reflecting on how the baby can see itself (*self*) through the mother's gaze, does Winnicott allude to face-to-face treatment – since he's not talking about a concrete gaze.

He even cites blind babies to make it clear that he is not talking about a concrete gaze, but more fundamentally about a subjective gaze, or more directly about the feelings of love, completeness and security that a mother can pass on to her child at a time when they feel indifferent from her.[21]

Obviously, reflecting on this idea of Winnicott's is not about recommending the couch for each and every case, not least because he always places himself as a mouldable object as an analyst, willing to make any changes to the *setting* that are in favour of the therapeutic aspect of the session. However, it is undeniable that thinking about the couch from the perspective that Winnicott understands it makes our theme more complex. If we were arguing that Ferenczi was concerned with welcoming the child who lives in the adult, perhaps we could say that Winnicott was concerned with welcoming the baby who lives in the adult (although the proposals of both are more complex than that).

Finally, there is also the posthumous publication *Holding and Interpretation: Fragments of an Analysis*,[22] in which Winnicott gives us the details of a clinical case in which the analysand had difficulties feeling good about himself and experiencing his true *self*. According to Winnicott, the analysand lacked the capacity for imagination and play, nor did he make spontaneous gestures or get excited about life in general. In a similar way to Ferenczi, Winnicott said that his job was to talk to the infant who lived inside the adult body. Specifically in relation to the couch, Winnicott intervenes by saying to the analysand: "The couch is me more than if I really hugged you",[23] which is closely linked to what was theorised earlier.

Also in this clinical case, Winnicott recounts several moments when the analysand put one foot on the floor, off the couch. As an analyst, he avoided interpreting the act as resistance (because, to a certain extent, it was), preferring to exalt the analysand's spontaneous gesture. This act (putting his foot down) would also be an attempt to "anticipate" the end of the session internally, since the analysand was afraid of being "sent away from the couch" by the analyst (by being surprised by the end of the session) – and would be preparing for a more direct contact with external reality (reality outside the session environment). This is very similar to what Ferenczi reported in *Restlessness at the End of the Analysis Session*,[24] which would reinforce a implicit affinity between the two authors – even though, as we have seen so far, the sum of Winnicott's contributions on the couch extends beyond Ferenczi.

Notes

1 Winnicott, (1954a) 2000a, p. 385.
2 Winnicott, (1947) 2000.
3 We will discuss the issues of the "skin that covers" again in Part I, Chapter 4, "Didier Anzieu's couch-skin".
4 Little, (1990) 1992.
5 Little, (1990) 1992, p. 46.
6 Little, (1990) 1992, pp. 95–96.

7 Maíra dos Santos Jaber (2013) works on my summarised statement in much more detail in her dissertation.
8 Winnicott, (1954b) 2000a.
9 Winnicott, (1954a) 2000a, p. 350.
10 Winnicott, (1954b) 2000a, p. 386.
11 About which he says: "There are no equal cases and there is a much freer exchange between therapist and patient than in pure psychoanalytic treatment" [Winnicott, (1971a) 1984a, p. 9].
12 Unlike other quotations taken from the book *From Paediatrics to Psychoanalysis*, published by Imago, this excerpt is taken from the Francisco Alves edition, since there is a difference in the translations, and this excerpt seems to choose more significant words, in line with what I'm thinking here [Winnicott, (1954a) 1993, p. 435].
13 Winnicott, (1962), 1984.
14 A term used by Winnicott himself [Winnicott, (1962) 1984, p. 435].
15 Winnicott, (1962) 1984, p. 152.
16 Winnicott, (1962) 1984, p. 155.
17 Winnicott, (1962) 1984, p. 154.
18 de Mattos (2016) states: "Classical interpretation is that which focuses on an unconscious desire related to a psychic conflict. It's important to clarify this because, as has already been pointed out, interpretation has taken on an expanded meaning."
19 Winnicott, (1962) 1984, p. 154.
20 Winnicott, (1967) 1975b, pp. 153–162.
21 In the text in question, Winnicott's main aim is to talk about how a mother's depression and the resulting difficulties in her investment in her baby would affect the baby's development.
22 Winnicott, (1972) 1986.
23 Winnicott, (1972) 1986.
24 Ferenczi, (1915) 2019.

Chapter 4

Didier Anzieu's skin couch

Didier Anzieu is known for his reflections on the self/non-self and the boundaries between the external and the internal. He theorises about the limits of the I-body and, starting from his conceptual metaphor of the I-skin, he thinks about how these limits fulfil functions in the constitution and containment of a psyche. Although brief, his contributions add to what we have been discussing from Winnicott onwards, at the same time as creating a kind of "bridge" to issues that will be raised in the following chapter.

In Anzieu's conception, the skin can be seen as a psychic envelope, a protective envelope for the internal world. The author established his conceptual metaphor – as he prefers to call it – on the basis of listening to sufferings arising from narcissistic wounds, closely linked to the "weakness or failure of the psychic envelope, a diffuse feeling of unease, a feeling of not inhabiting your life, of seeing your body and your thoughts work from the outside, of being the spectator of something that is and is not your own existence."[1] Let's see how his thinking affects the use of the couch.

In the book *I-Skin*[2] (*Le Moi-peau*) – more precisely in the chapter in which he tries to reflect on the I-skin as a thermal envelope – Anzieu tells us how, lying on the couch, an analysand regressed to primitive states, shivering and evoking the sensation of intense cold and sudden changes in temperature, evoking the sensations experienced when she was abused in her family during baths in her childhood. The analyst reports that

> It happened in many sessions that she reached an intermediate state between hallucination and depersonalisation: reality was no longer reality, her perception of things blurred, the three dimensions of space wavered; she herself continued to exist, but separated from her body, outside it.[3]

Through her analysis, the analysand's body evoked the suffering of yesteryear, reliving it. It would be through the work of analysis, being accompanied by the analyst in these moments of traumatic reliving, that she would be able to put into words what had been lived silently and denied by the environment around

DOI: 10.4324/9781003681212-6

her, her family. In her childhood, her feelings and the traumas she suffered were invalidated. Her skin was subjected to sudden changes in temperature, when sometimes she was subjected to boiling baths, and at other times to icy baths – in both cases, there was real torture disguised as care. The physical abuse, coupled with the invalidation of the traumatic experience, initially affected her skin but penetrated her inner psyche. It was in the company of the analyst that the analysand could validate her true suffering without it being called a "drama" (in the pejorative sense of the word), as her family used to call it. The revival in analysis would be in favour of a self-reconstruction.

Reflecting on "second skins", Anzieu states that, on many occasions, analysands, because of the regression in analysis, and the consequent revelations of "the destroyed and/or poorly connected parts of the Self",[4] end up reinforcing their "layers" during the intervals between sessions. He comments on analysands intensifying muscular exercises in order to reinforce layers between their self and the world, or keeping themselves warmer in the periods leading up to or following sessions – and that these analysands might also prefer to wrap themselves in blankets while lying on the couch – occasional comments that we could understand from what was being discussed in the previous chapter.

Anzieu reiterates that the use of the couch can evoke complaints that refer to failures in the maternal function. The analysand, when lying on the couch, could begin to complain of pain, bodily ailments and experiencing hypochondriacal feelings in order to "restore the function of continent skin not exercised by the mother or the human circle"[5] and, in the last resort, "self-infringing an envelope of suffering" along the lines of "I suffer, therefore I am", in order to ensure their existence through the experience of pain. These are situations that would certainly need to be handled appropriately by the psychoanalyst, although Anzieu doesn't delve into technical issues regarding how he would intervene in such moments.

Finally, it's important to point out that Didier Anzieu also dedicated himself to group psychoanalysis, so his work wasn't restricted to the couch. In an interview in 1986,[6] when asked about the possibility of giving up the couch in his work on individual analyses, Anzieu replied that, in certain cases, he gave the analysand freedom of choice, so that they could be face-to-face or even sitting on the floor, if they preferred. He prioritised "letting them adopt any spatial position that helps him communicate what he needs to say".[7]

With this, he also signalled that he would allow sessions to be conducted by phone call, since some analysands suffering from persecutory anxieties (or other types of excesses that would overwhelm their psyche) would benefit from them. This remote modality wouldn't surprise us in 2023, but it did surprise interviewer Gilbert Tarrab in 1986.

Furthermore, in the same interview, Anzieu ends up arguing that analysands who are more egoically damaged need to be looked at in the psychoanalytic session, which would agree with André Green's thinking, as will be seen below (Part I, Chapter 5, "André Green's couch: The dream model, other contributions and misreadings"). In this way, although part of Anzieu's thinking about the couch is connected to what was said by Winnicott, another part is connected to the need for the gaze defended by Green. With regard to his proposal for the analysand's "freedom of choice" (regarding the use of the couch), I would like to raise a question here, without wishing to answer it hastily: should the analysand's (conscious) preference be part of the analyst's theoretical-clinical thinking when choosing whether or not to use the couch?

Notes

1 Anzieu, 1989, p. 22.
2 Anzieu, 1989.
3 Anzieu, 1989, p. 22.
4 Anzieu, 1989.
5 Anzieu, 1989, p. 257.
6 Anzieu, 1990.
7 Anzieu, 1990, p. 59.

Chapter 5

André Green's couch

The dream model, other contributions and misreadings

André Green argues that the basis for the use of the couch lies in Freudian metapsychology, especially in *The Interpretation of Dreams*[1] because it understands the psychoanalytic frame and, consequently, the use of the couch, according to the dream model.

André Green's thinking, both about the function of the couch and its indication in analysis, is intrinsically based on the notion of the frame. Green is perhaps the author who has done the most to develop this theme, which has its high point in the important concept of *the analyst's internal frame*.

Therefore, it is important that, before we dedicate ourselves to thinking about the couch, I briefly present Green's conceptualisation of *the* frame, the *active matrix case*, as well as his proposal for *the analyst's internal frame* – since they corroborate his positions – and then go on to elucidate his thoughts on the function of the couch based on the dream model, and then point out a certain misreading on the part of Green with regard to its support in Winnicott's theorisations, especially with regard to the indication of face-to-face treatments because of the need to look.

It is therefore necessary to enter into a complex theoretical-clinical discussion, which will include clinical cases described by Green himself.

The beginning of this chapter will be dedicated to summarising, minimally, what the order of the frame will be, in order to then move on to think about the function of the couch in Green's thinking and discuss his positions.

* * *

The first conceptualisation of the frame was made in 1967 by José Bleger, who defined the *psychoanalytic situation* as the totality of the phenomena included in the therapeutic relationship between analyst and patient, indicating that this *psychoanalytic situation* constitutes a *process*. The frame, on the other hand, is "a '*non-process*', in the sense that it is the invariables that form the frame within which the *process* takes place".[2] Starting from José Bleger's conceptualisation, Green theorises the frame from two perspectives: (1) the *active matrix*, "made up of the patient's free association, attention and floating listening, marked by the analyst's benevolent neutrality, forming a *dialogical* pair in which analysis

DOI: 10.4324/9781003681212-6

takes root"; (2) the *case*, "made up of the number and duration of sessions, the periodicity of meetings, payment methods, etc.". "The active matrix is the jewel that the case contains."[3]

Each of these component elements of the frame would deserve to be discussed in detail if the focus of this book was to discuss them. However, it's enough to point out that, in a way, Bleger's "non-process" is similar, although not analogous, to what Green came to conceptualise as the *case of* the frame. However, according to both authors, the use of the couch would be included in what would be the order of this *case*, or of a "non-process", which serves to "frame" and which contains and aids the realisation of the psychoanalytic treatment.

Although we are not going to discuss in depth what all the elements of this "external" character of the frame consist of, which involves the contract, the number of sessions and/or any situation seen as of a concrete-external order, these issues will be presented throughout the book in some way, in the same way that it would be impossible to discuss the couch without mentioning free association, transference or other auxiliary concepts to listening. These are issues that have concerned clinical practice since Freud, even if they are not named from the conceptualisation of the frame.

In addition to thinking about the *active matrix* and the *frame case*, Green's thinking transcends them when he theorises about the *analyst's internal frame*, stating that it is:

> a figure from clinical thought to account for the analyst's necessary creation of an internal, intermediate space in which to sustain the analytical quality of communication when the patient is unable to recognise its metaphorical dimension, in which, due to the patient's limitations and attacks on his own functioning and on the treatment, the analyst must be able to invest the relationship as analytical (and not just interpersonal), postulating and sustaining the virtuality of the analytical process, for whom, for a long time, he must be the guarantor.
>
> What I'm talking about is that when the analytical frame doesn't work, it's possible to say that this is no longer a concept shared between the patient and the analyst. The frame comes from a notion internal to the analyst. It is the analyst who will have to assess what he or she hears in relation to a failure of representational functioning, which only he or she is able to perceive and understand. In these cases, we can't look for the unity of the analytical field on the patients, because we realise that their diversity implies very different forms of approach and even, on occasions, the renunciation of different formal aspects of the frame. In other words, the less the classic frame works, the more I am led to think that the unity of the psychoanalytic field can only be located in the analyst himself, in his clinical thinking.[4]

By emphasising the analyst's internal frame, Green opens doors for us to think about different ways of listening and intervening as psychoanalysts. As well as being an aid to psychoanalysts who practise their craft outside the consulting room, this notion reaffirms a profound ethical need for analytical practice. If the analyst is not sufficiently well analysed and does not have the conditions to ethically handle such a frame, they would be deviating from psychoanalytic practice. Let's take these points as implicit in everything that will be theorised until end of this book.

As for the "classic frame" and the rest of the discussion that concerns it, let's hold off on thinking about what Green will explore with regard to the use of the couch. I'll just point out here that, from the analyst's point of view, the couch being taken in its metaphorical function (which is a very important contribution from Green) does not exclude the possibility of the analysand taking it illusorily as the mother's body and its functions, as Winnicott advocated. In other words, the couch-object can be taken concomitantly from different angles depending on the internal world of each member of the analytic pair, since according to Winnicott's paradoxical thinking and for the development of a psyche, it is not important to define whether the object is created by the *infant* or presented to them by the external world,[5] the couch being a paradoxical object in which layers of functioning coexist and overlap.

At this point, it is also important to point out that it is from this perspective that Winnicott's thinking allows us to think beyond a dichotomy between what is internal and external, since it allows us to see the couch as an object that "lives" in the paradox between internal and external space – something that we will continue to discuss in the following chapters, especially in the second half of the book. Although examining the elements of the frame from the notions of internal and external – and the couch is understood as a component of the "external" order – is fundamental within Green's conceptualisations, it is not correlated to what we will work with from the etymology of *couch/diwan* in Part II of this book.

Later on, we will see that the etymological aspects of *couch/diwan* contain the notion of internal and external space at the same time, and this understanding will help us to think, for example, about clinical issues that involve working with what would be of the order of primary narcissism, taking into account the indication of the use of the couch.

* * *

For Green, the use of the couch is based on Freudian metapsychology. Its indication would be linked to what Freud theorised in *The Interpretation of Dreams*[6] and, from this point of view, the framing and indication of the couch would then be linked to the dream model.

> Although he didn't theorise in this way, Freud created the analytical frame along the lines of the dream. The reclining position, the suspension of motility, the delimitation of perception (because of the position of the analyst, outside the view of the patient, and the stable environment): all these

> factors produce a situation analogous to a dream, whose function is to allow (with the cooling of censorship) free association to unfold as close as possible to the primary processes.[7]
>
> The essential fact is the implicit homology between the dream model and the analytical frame model. Within the session, there is no closure of the perceptual pole, but the analyst offers the analysand a constant perception (the one seen from his couch) and places himself out of sight of the analysand. There is also no closure of the motor pole, but motricity is restricted by the lying position. It is between these two poles that the associative discourse takes place, with consciousness being conserved, but moral and intellectual censorship supposedly suspended, just as it is diminished within the dream. The agreement between the two models underpins the articulation between theory and practice.[8]

In fact, when describing the psychic apparatus in Chapter VII of *The Interpretation of Dreams*, Freud points out what Green would see as a prototype for the use of the couch in analysis. When we sleep, we all turn only to the internal world, reducing the receptivity of the perceptual pole (we close our eyes and "hallucinate") – a similar situation would occur with the motor pole (when we sleep, we are inert, which would help psychic events to unfold through dream work). This functioning would "expand" to the dynamics of the session, becoming a facilitator of free association, and also to all the internal mechanisms, such as displacement and condensation, reaching as far as the transferential field. The classic frame, which includes the use of the couch, favours the "virtuality" necessary for the analysis session, creating a space that is different from everyday life and "normal relationships".

Green points out differences in the framing of what he calls "classical psychoanalysis" and psychoanalytic psychotherapy. "Classical" psychoanalysis is defined by the use of the couch, a tool linked to the dream and neurosis model. Psychoanalytic psychotherapy, face-to-face (with eye contact), would be the model for severe, borderline cases.[9]

The frequency of sessions, for Green, does not determine what constitutes analysis (use of the couch) or psychotherapy (face-to-face), and there can be high or low frequency psychotherapy. In his conception, the indication for psychotherapy would be related to the patient's "more or less predictable intolerance of the analytic frame".[10] These intolerances of the classic frame would come from patients with "non-neurotic structures" and would challenge the analyst's clinical work. In order to deal with modes of framing that differ from "classical analysis", "sustain the metaphorising quality psychoanalytic communication"[11] and deal with the obstacles of listening and clinical intervention, Green relies on the notion of the psychoanalyst's *internal frame*, which was presented earlier. In his conception, it is the *internal frame* that allows the analyst to sustain the analytical work even in adverse situations or in situations beyond the classic frame. Therefore, it would be the analyst's internal frame that would sustain changes of frame, such as giving up the couch and working face-to-face.

In view of this, I believe it is important to problematise the indication of face-to-face, taking into account Green's own theorising about the *framing structure*, as will be done below.

* * *

Despite Green's important theoretical constructions, I believe it is important to point out a contradiction in his argument that may go unnoticed by the reader. This misreading refers to how the author draws on Winnicott's thought to articulate the indication of face-to-face in a way that is incongruent with his own, Green's, but also Winnicott's, statements. In spite of Winnicott's statement about carrying out a "modified analysis" when necessary,[12] this is not the point that Green sought to explore in his arguments.

In an interview with Fernando Urribarri, Green defends the idea of the "good-enough mother" as the founder of the *framing structure*:

> What do *hold* and *handle* mean for the baby being held? What does it mean? Well, precisely: a framing structure. When you're separated from your mother, it's not the memory of her face or her smile that matters. What counts are the traces of the frame that the contact of her body represented. Mother's face and smile can disappear or be replaced. The frame remains.[13]

Green quotes Winnicott to emphasise that the frame provided by being in the mother's arms, lap and body is more important than the unique configuration of her features and eye contact with her. However, in the same interview, he says that, in serious cases, it is necessary to change the frame and start accepting face-to-face treatment because of the importance of the gaze.[14] Well then, if Green claims that the bodily framing within the mother's arms is more important than the gaze, why does his clinical justification for face-to-face work rely primarily on the gaze?

This is also curious, since Winnicott's text on the gaze, *The Mother's and Family's Role in the Child's Development as a Mirror*[15] (which does not, at any point, question the use of the couch), is not used by Green to theoretically articulate face-to-face work.

There is a contradiction, because in this interview with Urribarri, to articulate the idea of face-to-face care to the detriment of the couch, Green quotes Winnicott's text "Hate in Countertransference" (1947) and, to defend the same point, in his book *Guidelines for Contemporary Psychoanalysis*,[16] he also quotes Winnicott – this time, the text "Metapsychological and Clinical Aspects of Regression within the Psycho-Analytical Set-Up" (1954).[17] An even greater incongruity, since not only does Winnicott not make any indication in favour of switching from the couch to face-to-face, but in both of the texts cited by Green, he emphasises the paradox of the couch being/representing the "mother's body" and the possibility of analysis taking place on the basis of this understanding, as we saw earlier. Therefore, in order to defend the face-to-face in non-neurotic cases, he used the texts in which Winnicott demonstrates an interesting use of the couch in non-neurotic cases.

It is through two contradictions, readings that are contrary to Winnicott's writing, that Green articulates the face-to-face and the importance of the gaze in the *setting*. If Green himself says that the mother's body/setting is more important than the gaze, why would he prioritise the gaze? What's even stranger is that he does this on the basis of Winnicott's texts in which he talks about the couch as the mother's body and tries to elucidate the complexity that the use of the couch can have.

Despite this, Green's misreading does not diminish the importance of his thinking, nor the importance of problematising the gaze as a possible aid in treatment. However, if Green remained faithful to his own assertion that the frame/body of the mother is more important than the gaze, relying on Winnicott's theorising to defend a practice, Green could state that the "borderline" analysand should lie on the couch – because this frame would refer to the mother's body (*framing structure*) – and the couch would be/represent[18] the *holding* and *handling*, more fundamental than the gaze (according to Green's own assertion).

In this sense, in order to emphasise the importance of the concreteness of the gaze, it seems to me that Green would have to look for another conceptual basis to defend the face-to-face, and not the ones that he sought precisely in Winnicott's work.

* * *

To continue the discussion, it's important to mention a few more of Green's considerations regarding the use or non-use of the couch.

In the interviews with Fernando Urribarri, André Green tells us that he decided to recommend the use of the couch for patients who until then had been seen by other analysts in face-to-face treatments. Green[19] comments that, in his practice, he would see these patients fall "into a kind of anobjectal desert", into a "mental desertification syndrome", which he considers to be an inversion of the postulates of the analytic situation, since Freud would have thought of it as favouring free association and allowing oneiric functioning to come as close as possible to oneiric processes. Let's look in detail at how Green thinks about the situation:

> what happens here, with the cases I've described, is that instead of obtaining an associative unfettering, we see a withdrawal on the part of the individual, like a snail closing in on its shell. Of course, one could reflect and say that, in these cases, perhaps the analyst is experienced as a potential aggressor.

> But that's not what the patients themselves feel. Their feeling is that there is no one. The object desert is absolute ... Everything is empty. Nothing makes sense, nothing connects. In these circumstances, it can be assumed that we are dealing with terror.[20]

The first question we might ask is why he would indicate the couch, given that he himself would be advocating face-to-face in such cases. However, beyond this question, we can see how this passage from the interview – and also its sequence – makes it clear that Green believes that the analyst's direct "non-vision" would mean for the analysand that the analyst-object has withdrawn (is absent). An understanding that, in fact, would be completely true if the analyst really withdrew psychically from the situation, seeing the couch only as an instrument linked to "associative unfurling", in which the analyst must remain silent, waiting for this unfurling to take place.

Green's position takes into account what he himself sees as the doing of analysis, and he is very specific about this. His reaffirmative position, over the years, against a series of research studies, above all those linked to observations of babies,[21] and advocating in favour of a "purely clinical" psychoanalysis – pointing out the "dangers" of these observations for psychoanalysis – ends up ignoring part of the work with the primitive in the *setting*.[22]

Could it be that we are speaking of an analyst who would not tolerate the primitive, helpless "infant" that lives within the analysand from emerging on the couch, and therefore would avoid this type of approach? If the answer were affirmative, it would indeed be fair and advisable for Green to avoid the couch; after all, the analyst must, ethically, feel at least minimally comfortable, in psychic terms, in order to support any indication, whatever it may be.

Following the interview, Green argues that it's as if the "primary objects have never allowed themselves to be transformed. In order for the 'transformational object' to help transform, it must begin by allowing itself to be transformed". This is a very important phrase and one that, in my view, is closely linked to the role of the analyst. However, before commenting on Green's passage, it is necessary to introduce the concept he borrows.

The concept of a transformational object comes from Christopher Bollas. In Part I, Chapter 7, "Christopher Bollas and the evocative couch", I will go into this author's thinking in more depth, although it's necessary to focus a little here on the transformational. The transformational experience is an aesthetic experience of being transformed by the object relationship. Let's understand the initial prototype of the baby being transformed by the mother object:

> Before the mother was personalised for the baby as a total object, she functioned as a region or as a source of transformation. And since the baby's own nascent subjectivity is almost completely an experience of the integrations of the ego (cognitive, libidinal, affective), the first object is identified with the alterations in the state of the ego. With the baby's growth and

increasing self-confidence, the relationship with the mother changes from "mother as the other who alters the self" to a person who has their own life and their own needs.[23]

If we take Bollas's thinking in its full scope, we will see that, on the one hand, he speaks of the primary transformational object, as in the example cited; but, on the other hand, he also seeks to reflect on object relations with transformational potential that occur in other spheres of life, especially in the analytic space. Thus, for Bollas, the analyst is an object for use by the analysand, endowed with transformational potential. If Green states that, for a transformation to occur in the other, one must first allow oneself to be transformed, he is speaking of the function the analyst must (or should) exercise in an analysis. In other words, the analyst needs to be open to being transformed in the relationship with the other (the analysand) so that this analysand may, in turn, also be transformed.

Therefore, if we return to Ferenczi and the importance of the adult adapting to the needs of the child (and not the other way round) in favour of a healthy development of the psyche, we have new questions to ask: Who can't adapt to whom? Would the analyst who recommends the couch for cases of "mental desertification" not be adapting to the needs of the analysand and be recommending face-to-face therapy? Or is the analyst who recommends face-to-face not adapting to the analysand's need to regress in session? In these cases, shouldn't the analyst adapt to the process of regression and the "anobjectality" referred to by Green, making themselves available as a primitive and transformational object of use for the analysand?

These questions are fundamental, because it can be misleading to think that making use of face-to-face means adapting to the analysand's needs. Should their need to regress to these anobject stages in an analysis be ignored? I repeat: I don't intend to invalidate or think of the indications of the face-to-face as less important or ineffective, because, in fact, it will always depend on the conditions of the analyst and the analysand in question; but I believe it is fundamental that this discussion should take into account the highest complexity, without falling into the risks of systematisation based on pathological typologies.

Furthermore, being face-to-face with someone has never been a guarantee of an effective and profound "presence"; that's why we can't apply the notions of absence and presence only through the visual prism, since it can be felt in other ways; for example, through the constancy of the analyst's voice or even through breathing and bodily noises, since the work with the primitive is not necessarily or primarily based on the association of the words spoken by the analysand, but also through what their body says.

All this discussion makes it clear that if, for Winnicott, the use of the couch is not synonymous with classical technique, for Green it is. Perhaps an in-depth study and development of Green's *work on the negative* and his theorising on the function of the presence and absence of the object for psychic constitution could lead us to a reflection closer to the one we see in Winnicott about the couch. Technical proposals, if thought of from the perspective of the paradox of the absence-presence of the object, which are intrinsic characteristics of the couch – due to the fact that the gaze is cut off at the same time as there is the presence of the analyst's voice, together with all of Winnicott's comments about the couch as a body – could also be thought of by Green for serious cases. In the text *The Intuition of the Negative in Playing and Reality*, from the book *André Green at the Squiggle Foundation*,[24] a compilation of lectures given by Green aimed at an interlocution between his thinking and Winnicott's, Green states: "It is important to experience it, the object being outside of omnipotent control"[25] and adds that:

> imaginative elaboration is closely linked to absence. I have already said on another occasion that the psyche is the relationship between two bodies, one of which is absent. The originality of Winnicott's contribution to this problem is that he opened up a way out of the traditional dilemma of emphasising absence or, conversely, presence. What he did was to consider – once again – the point between meeting (presence) and separation (absence). This view enriched the theory of symbolism by providing a dynamic view of it, emphasising the moment in which the parts were separated or united again – hence the corollary: the object is found (as opposed to lost) and created (as opposed to perceived). This implies an entirely new view of the relationship between representation (i.e. memory) and perception (i.e. consciousness).[26]

The question of absence and imaginative elaboration mentioned by Green is extremely important and will be central to Part II of this book, so nothing that can be developed here will reach the complexity that we will discuss later. As for the rest, it seems self-explanatory to me. I'd like to emphasise how much Green talks about the importance of the absence of the object for this created being, or rather, the paradox of presence-absence – precisely the paradox that Winnicott's use of the couch was designed to accommodate, with the marked presence of the analyst, albeit without the excess of the face-to-face gaze. Absence (and here we should think of the absence of the gaze) as a precondition for representation is a Freudian precept incorporated and repeated by Green and one that could also be used to articulate the use of the couch in those clinical cases in which the analyst, Green, wants to establish representational chains where there are none. Isn't this, in a reflection by Green himself, the justification for the use of the couch also in analyses involving more damaged psyches?

Although Green is confronting his own position and his indication of face-to-face for borderline cases, it is possible to find clinical vignettes in his work in which these treatments are taking place on the couch.

In the book *Life Narcissism, Death Narcissism*,[27] when portraying narcissistic disorders, Green states that some analysands "lie down in a stereotyped way, not allowing themselves to change position or make any kind of movement". On the couch, the "body would speak" viscerally, through bowel sounds, vasomotor reactions, sweating, sensations of cold or heat, these expressions coming from a bad relationship established between the mother (and her libidinal tendencies) and the baby (the analysand). In this case, Green describes the analysand's fragility and even the analyst's countertransference feelings of repulsion towards the analysand – but we don't know about his interventions, since his account ends at this point, without Green elaborating on them. However, the clinical phenomena he presents are similar to those described by Winnicott, who, on a technical level, would at first show acceptance (as long as it was genuine) for the manifestations of this "regressed baby" (Green himself uses the term baby), since we are dealing with a person with narcissistic failures.

It would be from this angle that the couch would serve as an aid to proper *handling* and *holding*, at the same time as protecting the analysand from the invasion of the gaze and even from the countertransferential feelings of rejection mentioned by Green. In *The New Psychoanalytic Clinic and Freud's Theory: Fundamental Aspects of Private Madness*,[28] Green recalls, evoking Winnicott again: "in borderline cases, the analyst does not represent the mother: he is the mother".

In Green's book *On Private Madness*,[29] there are more descriptions of clinical situations that take place on the couch. Although he discusses the extent to which there are situations that "escape" and "act" outside the classical frame, such as the occurrence of somatic discharges and emotional overflows linked failures of narcissistic functions, it is interesting that – in this and other books – many of his clinical descriptions take place on the couch.

In general terms, we see Green describing borderline situations from the point of view of their tendency towards fusional regression and object dependence, even announcing that the analyst's function (as object) would be to help this integration.[30] This theoretical exposition, when transposed to the clinic, wouldn't lead us to think about the function of the couch and the very notions of body *and container* (an expression he adopted from Bion)? Wouldn't the point at which the analysand with serious suffering is regressed be the moment when the analyst's libidinising intervention could potentially help them most in their integrative processes? There are no easy answers.

Referring to the proposals of Green, Winnicott and many other psychoanalysts, Jaime M. Lutenberg[31] states that when the analyst is seen face-to-face, this helps him to control the "psychopathological regression" that can occur during the session. The term "psychopathological regression" appears only once in his text, in a vague way, but I'm concerned about its use. It might be interesting to think about it, but not without first making it clear that, despite his reference to pathology, when Lutenberg describes the phenomenon, it is essentially no different from the regression to dependence proposed by Winnicott, since all of Lutenberg's theorising is based on an initial, fusional moment between baby and mother in the constitution of the psyche. From this, questions can be raised that problematise the terminology in order to help us think about the clinic: Should a "psychopathological regression" be avoided in a psychoanalytic session? Isn't one of the functions of the analytical process precisely that psychopathology lodges itself in the *setting* in order to be treated? Isn't it a function of analysis that psychopathology expresses itself more and more in the *setting*, so that it gradually reduces its impact in "real life" (outside the consulting room)?

The theoretical-clinical contradiction we find in Green only makes it clear how complex and diverse the positions around the possible uses and non-uses of the couch can be. It is notable that Green considers the concreteness of the gaze to be important in the cases mentioned, even though his theoretical justification may allude to other paths. James M. Lutenberg,[32] taking into account the propositions regarding the psychotic and non-psychotic parts of the personality theorised by Bion, and evoking the word *play*, leaves it up to his analysands to choose the way they "need" the session to be conducted. Thus, an analysand can predominantly lie down on the couch, but get up, walk around the room and sit down in front of the analyst, according to their bodily and internal needs. For him, it would be the oscillation between his psychotic and non-psychotic parts that would determine how the analysand would occupy the psychoanalytic space. William I. Grossman,[33] when comparing a borderline case presented by Green to another presented by Kernberg, comments that the way in which treatment is conducted also differs due to gradations. Green's case[34] was treated on the couch, while Kernberg's was conducted outside of it, in an institution and with a much greater load of destructiveness. These are undoubtedly important arguments.

Green's constant reaffirmation,[35] differentiating psychoanalysis from psychotherapy on the basis of an external frame – even though he makes it clear that he doesn't disdain the second term – sound problematic to me terminologically, as their conception restricts the term *psychoanalysis* to the so-called "classical" frame. We are currently talking about psychoanalysis 80 years after Freud's death.

And, taking this into account, can we still say that psychoanalysis would be the "classical" model, while the "rest" would be psychotherapy? If we focus only on our theme (which is the use of the couch), we must ask ourselves: Can't we think about its use beyond what Freud initially thought?

Green's great and unequivocal theoretical contribution seems to me to be about the *analyst's internal frame*, because it is this concept that allows us to listen and intervene psychoanalytically in "any situation". If an analyst is listening and intervening from his or her psychoanalytic internal frame, couldn't we say that this analyst is being an analyst and is working in a process of analysis, whatever the particularity of this work? Certainly, yes – just as Green also points out that the external frame and the couch do not guarantee that there is a process of psychoanalysis. The analysand (including a neurotic) may be resisting analysis and working with it from their Unconscious; however, if the psychoanalyst is working in this direction, I don't think that changing the term psychoanalysis to another one will help us.

I don't think that an analyst should "abandon" psychoanalysis within himself (his internal frame) and fail to take it into account in any possible modification that his work may have. "Modified analysis", as Winnicott proposes, is more unspecific and perhaps more appropriate. In a way, all analyses are "modified", none is the same the other. More controversy could be raised about the term psychotherapy, since the notion of therapy is present in Freud's work. Freud, above all, works for a "cure", even if this can be considered an unattainable ideal. The aforementioned Winnicott and many others also do not dissociate therapy as inherent to psychoanalytic work.

But let's leave this controversial chapter aside for a moment and continue to consider the contributions of other authors, without forgetting to emphasise how Green's model of the dream, transposed to an understanding of the function of the couch, is a fundamental contribution clinical practice.

Notes

1 Freud, (1900) 2019.
2 Bleger, 1988, p. 311.
3 Green, 2008, p. 54.
4 Urribarri, 2013, p. 121.
5 Winnicott tells us about an illusion of omnipotence, a creative omnipotence, in which, in a primary moment, from the baby's point of view, it makes no difference whether the object is presented to him or created by him – it doesn't matter whether it was offered to him by his mother or whether he created it himself. The good-enough mother enables the baby to experience omnipotence, the experience of "creating" the external reality that it offers him [Winnicott, (1953) 1975a; (1969) 1975c; (1971a) 1975d].
6 Freud, (1900) 2019.
7 Green, Urribarri, 2019, p. 80.
8 Green, 2004, p. 23
9 This idea that differentiates psychoanalysis, its classic model, with the use of the couch, from psychotherapy (face-to-face and serious cases) is a thought that runs through Green's work and is present in more than one of the interviews that make up the book *From Clinical Thought to the Contemporary Paradigm*, 2019), as well as being found on pages 38–43 of the book *Orientations for a Contemporary Psychoanalysis* (2008) – books that aim, in a way, to "synthesise" the author's theoretical-clinical thought (Green, 2008a; Green and Urribarri, 2019).
10 Green, 2008a, p. 49.
11 Urribarri, Green, 2010, p. 40.
12 Although Green intended to make this point, we saw in Part I, Chapter 3, "The couch-body of Donald Woods Winnicott", how Winnicott's intention was not to advocate treatment, but to explore ways of intervening (still on the couch) that would transcend classical interpretation.
13 Green, Urribarri, 2019, pp. 64–65.
14 Green, Urribarri, 2019, p. 70.
15 Winnicott, (1967) 1975b, pp. 153–162.

16 Green, 2008a, p. 49.
17 Precisely the texts in which Winnicott writes about regression to dependence on the couch.
18 According to the paradox of being/representing, present in Winnicott's theorising.
19 Green, Urribarri, 2019, p. 83.
20 Green, Urribarri, 2019, p. 84.
21 Green, 1979a, pp. 27–47.
22 In this respect, we cannot deny the importance of observation, much of Freud's theoretical construction is based on it. For example, when Freud observes and interprets his grandson's "Fort/Da game" [Freud, (1920) 2010].
23 Bollas, 2015, p. 63.
24 Originally edited by Jan Abram in 2000, it is derived from lectures given by Green in the United Kingdom and is a compilation by the Squiggle Foundation [see Green, (2000a) 2003].
25 Green, (2000b) 2003, p. 63.
26 Green, (2000a) 2003, p. 65.
27 Green, (1988), p. 143.
28 Green, 1994, p. 86.
29 Green, (1986) 2005.
30 Green, (1986) 2005, p. 38.
31 Lutenberg, 2007, p. 102.
32 Lutenberg, 2007, pp. 102–103.
33 Grossman, 2007.
34 Published as *The Central Phobic Position: A New Formulation of the Free Association Method* [Green, 2000b, 2002].
35 Green, 2011.

Chapter 6

Thomas Ogden and privacy on the couch

Thomas Ogden[1] reminds us that Freud's use of the couch was not only theoretically based on facilitating the analysand's free association, although we know that it was. Ogden emphasises that its use was linked to the fact that Freud couldn't bear to be observed during his listening process.[2] This reminder is relevant because Ogden wants to emphasise the analyst's need for privacy in carrying out his work. In his, Ogden's, view, the analyst needs privacy to listen, to surrender to the flow of the analysand's unconscious thoughts, and visual contact between the analyst and the analysand would impair the analyst's listening.

In this sense, by returning to Freud, Ogden stresses the importance of using the couch not only for the analysand, but also for the analyst, as he believes that visual contact would damage the privacy of the pair and their relationship as a whole. Despite this, his conception of the couch and of abstaining from the gaze is not intended to be dictatorial.

After all, it would be enough for the analysand to turn his head to see the analyst, as his clinical cases clearly demonstrate.[3]

> In an effort to create a space for dreaming, I sit behind the couch while the patient lies on it. I explain to each patient at the beginning of an analysis that their use of the couch affords me the privacy I need to think in a way different from how I think in face-to-face conversation. I add that the patient will likely find this true for themselves as well.[4]
>
> I would add that the analysand may also find that this way of working allows them to experience their own thoughts in a different direction to their usual way of thinking, feeling and experiencing physical sensations. The fact that I introduce the use of the couch by emphasising my own need, as well as that of the analysand, for an area of privacy, a psychological space (both literally and metaphorically) in which to think and generate experiences, represents an important statement to the patient about my conception of the analytic method and the overlapping of our roles in it.

DOI: 10.4324/9781003681212-8

> In what has been outlined so far, it is implicit that I consider the circumstances necessary for both analyst and patient to be able to achieve the state of *reverie* as a necessary condition for conducting the analysis.[5]

Each member of the analytic pair would have the right to their own privacy, their own space, without being invaded by the other's gaze. It would be from this space that both would be better able to devote themselves to their craft: free association and floating attention, respectively. Ogden argues that privacy from the other's gaze leads the analyst and the analysand to their own states of *reverie*, a prerequisite for the process of analysis.

Reverie could be thought of as akin to a "dream state".[6] We can understand it as what emerges in the analyst's mind to help him or her build hypotheses about what the analysand is unable to communicate formally.

> For me, *reverie*, waking dream, is paradigmatic of the clinical experience of intuiting the psychic reality of a moment in analysis. To enter a state of *reverie*, which in the analytic setting is always part of an intersubjective phenomenon, the analyst must engage in an act of self-renunciation. By self-renunciation, I mean the act of allowing oneself to be more than just oneself in order to create a psychological space in which analyst and patient can enter into a shared state of intuition and jointly share a disturbing psychic reality that the patient is unable to face alone. The analyst doesn't seek to achieve *reverie* any more than he seeks to achieve intuition. *Reverie* and intuition come, if they come at all, without effort, "spontaneously".[7]

According to Ogden, the analytic structure is designed to enable "overlapping states of *reverie*",[8] a third space of overlap/intersection between the *reverie of* the analysand and that of the analyst, called the *intersubjective analytic third.* His proposal of overlapping states derives from Winnicott's thinking:[9] there is what is private, what is the other's, and space shared between the two; but it also takes into account Bion's container/contained relationship. There is what can only be experienced within each one (analysand and analyst), and there is something that can be experienced in this third instance, permeated by parts shared psychically by each member of the analytic pair.

> The structure (for example, the use of the couch) and the psychoanalytic technique (for example, the method of free association used by both the analysand and the analyst) are designed to increase each participant's ability to reach a state of mind in which they can access the ongoing unconscious conversation with themselves that takes the form of a dream during sleep and a *reverie* in waking life. The analyst's state of *reverie* involves a withdrawal from the logic, demands and distractions of external reality, which would be like the experience of the "darkness" of sleep (the isolation

> of the mind from the glare of consciousness) – a darkness in which the dream, a continuous psychic event, becomes perceptible. As Freud said (1916), "I have to blind myself artificially in order to concentrate … on a dark point". The analyst's state of *reverie* is his waking dream or his sleeping vigil, a state in which he glimpses into the shadows of the productions of the unconscious. As one matures as an analyst, one's eyes become more readily "adapted to the darkness".[10]

Ogden defines how using the couch (with the analyst sitting behind it, out of the analysand's field of vision) favours the conditions in which analyst and analysand can each have enough privacy to enter their own *reverie* states,[11] which sometimes leads the analyst to access sensations and feelings that are not exactly his own, but come from the shared experience with his analysand through the analytic third.[12]

Stating that it is difficult to understand the logic of working face-to-face with an analysand,[13] Ogden believes that even if there is a reason to carry out a treatment with a low frequency, the couch should be used. Giving up the couch as an instrument because of the impossibility of a high frequency treatment would be unjustified and even harmful. For him, the quality of the encounter depends, among other factors, on the analyst being in the best possible listening condition – an issue closely linked to the idea that the analyst needs a private space (for himself) to listen to the other. In his view, the couch would be a facilitator in any circumstance, although he asserts that there are times when it can become too frightening for the analysand, and pressuring them to use it would be anti-therapeutic.

It is necessary to put into context that the immense importance given by Ogden to the question of the privacy of the analyst and the analysand is not only related to the use of the couch. That would be just one facet of his thinking about privacy in the session. Thus, Ogden justifies the use of the couch from his understanding of privacy and, in the same way, justifies the fundamental rule of an analysis. He advocates reformulating the initial proposal that the analysand "must" say everything that comes into his mind to one in which he "has the right" to say everything that comes into his mind. Thus, Ogden operates a shift in meaning in which what is important is not the "duty" to open one's mind to the analyst, but that the analysand has the "right" to tell everything that comes to mind, without judgement on the part of the analyst.[14]

From this perspective, the analysand can keep to himself something that, for whatever reason, he wants to keep private. They have the right, together with the analyst, to bare to the highest degree possible, according to their psychic conditions, but they don't necessarily "have to" do so, since one of their sufferings can come from an invasion of their private space.

What I have described so far would be fundamental in the treatment of the most varied psychopathologies, but it is important to dedicate ourselves once again to the discussion about the use of the couch beyond neurotic suffering, as has been articulated in previous chapters. Although Ogden's clinical cases reinforce the use of the couch as an ally in the work related to sexual and oedipal issues[15] in neuroses, let's look at some cases in which Ogden's statements become fundamental for working with patients who are more psychically vulnerable, experiencing narcissistic suffering.

In a clinical excerpt,[16] evoking Winnicott's theory and clinic, Ogden recounts an analysand's first session. In this case, even though it was her first meeting with the analyst, as soon as the analysand entered the consulting room, she went to the couch. Lying down, she reports suffering from panic attacks, not being able to work and not being able to fulfil her role as a mother. And, like someone who doesn't attach much importance to the subject, she ends up mentioning the death of her mother months before.

In his sessions with this analysand, Ogden felt intrusive when the analysand made any noise other than just breathing, claiming to have "learned to say practically nothing" in his sessions. "Even moving in the armchair was experienced by the patient as if I had slapped her."[17] His understanding was that the analysand was also making a lot of effort to tolerate being with the analyst.

A continuous sharing of silence and breathing together in the space of the session made Ogden remember when he had to attune the rhythm of his breathing to that of his son – when the little one was three years old – in order to calm him down and get him to sleep. One night with him, Ogden had a very intense dream that his wife and his son had disappeared. Ogden's *reverie* implies that it is this overwhelming feeling of the disappearance of a loved one that is at play in the session.

Ogden's dream would be a presentation (within himself) of what his son might be feeling. And, consequently, what would the analysand be feeling?[18] Are we talking about the analysand's need to feel cosy, united (by breathing) with the primary object? Are we talking about the need to feel alive? Beyond a discussion about the couch, this passage demonstrates Ogden's clinical work based on his *reverie*, and how his listening is intertwined with his propositions. He points out that this clinical situation deals with not only a psychological experience, but also a physical one, in developing his thinking on the basis of Winnicott, he states:

> *Holding* is an ontological concept that Winnicott uses to explore the specific qualities of the experience of being alive at different stages of development, as well as the changing intrapsychic-interpersonal means by which the sense of continuity of being is sustained over time.[19]
>
> As the baby grows, the function of *holding* shifts from safeguarding the tissue of the baby's going-on-being to sustaining, over time, the modes of being alive that are more related to the object. One of these later forms of *holding* involves providing a place (a psychological state) in which the baby (or patient) can organize themselves.[20]

Ogden's reflections point towards conceiving a bodily dimension of the couch (associated with holding),[21] while at the same time also converging on the idea of approaching its use through a dream model – albeit a different one from the model described by Green.

In the book *The Primitive Edge of Experience*,[22] Ogden brings up the case of Mr R, also treated on the couch, where he, Mr R, felt he couldn't think or speak in the sessions. The analysand experienced himself as completely empty and, although he longed to be in analysis, he experienced it as terrifying. Nevertheless, according to Ogden, little by little,

> Mr R. unconsciously managed to create a sensory basis for himself by filling in what he later called "holes" both in himself (his inability to think or speak) and in the analytic relationship (which he experienced as non-existent) by focusing intently on a rectangular shape that he distinguished in the pattern of lines and texture on the ceiling above the sofa. These "holes" were later understood to be partly derivative of the "holes" in his early experience of the mother-baby relationship, due to his mother's deep postnatal depression, for which she was quickly hospitalised. His mother told him, during the period of R.'s analysis, that she had held him as a baby only when "absolutely necessary". He was left to cry in his cot for hours on end while his mother hid in her bedroom.[23]

This excerpt reaffirms the possibility of understanding the function of the couch as a *holding*, at the same time as there is a projection of the analysand's internal "holes" onto the external world (the ceiling and its textures). Ogden presents us with the possibility of thinking about the "creation of a sensory base for oneself" when this is psychically necessary. The feeling of terror the analysand experienced while lying on the couch was, first and foremost, that of being abandoned in his crib; however, his analytic experience shows us that the reliving of abandonment – arising from the transferential experience and the use of the couch – holds transformative potential. The "holes" in the ceiling become an opportunity to encounter his own and to "fill them in" as corporeal surfaces.

In the book in which this and other cases are found, Ogden was engaged in the theoretical development of the autistic–contiguous position, an addition to Klein's depressive and paranoid–schizoid positions. This position would have more primitive, pre-symbolic and sensory characteristics. The defences generated in this autistic–contiguous mode "are directed toward re-establishing the continuity of the bounded sensory surface and the ordered rhythmicity upon which the initial integrity of the self rests,"[24] a quest to restore one's bodily cohesion. According to Ogden, twirling one's hair, tapping one's feet, stroking one's lips or earlobe, seeking symmetrical and geometric shapes in the ceiling or wall as reference points, or using one's fingers to trace shapes on the wall beside the couch are self-soothing activities of autistic forms that live within all of us, to a greater or lesser degree. The analytic hour would also serve the purpose of building or rebuilding the edges of the self.

Other interesting cases, found in the same book, corroborate his hypotheses, such as that of the female analysand[25] who had skin problems – especially on her face – and suffered from insomnia. At a certain point, she ended up sleeping through an entire session following an intervention by Ogden that is difficult to summarize briefly here, but was surely welcoming and very well articulated in relation to what had been experienced in the session. According to his account of the case, she achieved sufficient internal safety to allow herself to drift into sleep, to rest. Ogden's understanding is that she made use of the analyst and the couch as a second skin.

In a chapter devoted to thinking about the feeling of being alive in one's own body, from the book *Conversations at the Frontier of Dreaming*,[26] Ogden offers the example of a man who had been molested in childhood and who, at times, would become disorganized and roll from side to side on the couch. The continuity of the analytic work led, at a certain point in the treatment, to this man feeling that "his body was there",[27] stating that he could not recall ever having felt that he possessed a body before. An internal process had taken place for him to be able to take ownership of his body. After an emblematic session, in which he felt fully that he was the owner of his own body, he came to the following session saying that he would like to lie on the couch and sleep, reporting that the night before he had dreamt he was the analyst of a baby, but that, at the end of the dream, after understanding some of the figures that had appeared in it, he lay down beside the baby – in its crib – being observed (cared for) in a fraternal way by a figure representing Ogden. We could not go into the details of the dream, not least because I present only a summary, but it certainly speaks of an analytic process and of the couch/crib as a secure space, of rest and tranquillity, for development. The point is that, through this clinical case, Ogden seeks to highlight the work of reconnecting what may have been split (mind and body) as a product of trauma, and the couch plays a central role in this connection/reconnection with oneself as a whole.

> However one defines analysis, it seems essential to include in this definition the attempt to generate and experience the unconscious analytic third to foster a state of *reverie* through which analyst and analysand can perceive the "flow" of the shared (and yet individually experienced) unconscious construction. The analytic endeavour is best defined not by its format (such as the frequency of sessions), but by its substance, which involves the analysis of transference–countertransference (including anxiety/defence), as these phenomena take form in the experience and interpretation of the analytic third.[28]

In Ogden's clinical conception, "the most fundamental purpose of the analytic relationship is to help the analysand make psychological changes that enable him to live his life in a more fully human manner".[29] What we have seen from his proposals about privacy in analysis and the materiality of the couch as an aid to treatment, combined with the rest of his theory and technique, is fundamental for thinking about the psychoanalytic practice and the ways in which we can conceive the use of the couch.

Notes

1 Ogden, 2013, pp. 101–124.
2 "I cannot bear to be stared at by other people for eight hours (or more) a day, since while I am listening to the patient, I also give myself over to the current of my unconscious thoughts," says Freud in *On Beginning the Treatment* (1913a) 1996. See Chapter 1, "Sigmund Freud's couch-reminiscence".
3 In *Subjects of Analysis*, Ogden also mentions the act of the analysand turning their head to look at the analyst (Ogden, 1994, pp. 88, 158).
4 Ogden, 2016, p. 2.
5 Ogden, 2013, pp. 108–109.
6 *Reverie* is one of the translations of the German *Tagtraum*, used by Freud.
7 Ogden, 2016, pp. 79–80.
8 Ogden, 2013, p. 110.
9 Ogden supports his idea with a passage from Winnicott. He argues that treatment takes place in the space of overlap/intersection between the play areas of the analysand and the analyst. The word used by Winnicott is *overlap*. Winnicott's original phrase is "psychotherapy takes place in the overlap of two areas of playing, that of the patient and that of the therapist" (Winnicott, 1971a, p. 38). See Winnicott, 1975, 2019; 1971b.
10 Cf. Ogden, 2002, pp. 5–6. Freud's quote is taken from his correspondence with Lou Andreas-Salomé [Freud (1916), 1966].
11 Ogden, 2013, p. 111.
12 Ogden, 2016, p. 24.
13 Ogden, 2013, p. 112.
14 Ogden, 2013, p. 116.
15 In *Conversations at the Frontier of Dreaming* (2002, pp. 34–36), Ogden talks about sexual and Oedipal aspects in relation to the couch.
16 Ogden, 2005a, pp. 95–96.
17 Ogden, 2005a, p. 121; Ogden, 2005b, p. 95.
18 Beyond considering Ogden's views on countertransference and *reverie*, we might also think in terms of mechanisms of projective identification.
19 Ogden, (2005a) 2010, p. 122.
20 Ogden, (2005b) 2010, p. 125.
21 Even if this is not the author's theoretical proposal.
22 Ogden, 1989.
23 Ogden, 1989a, p. 37.
24 Ogden, 1989a, p. 379.
25 Ogden, 1989a, pp. 71–72.
26 Ogden, 2002.
27 Ogden, 2022a, p. 166.
28 Ogden, 2013, p. 112.
29 Ogden, 2013, p. 105.

Chapter 7

Christopher Bollas and the evocative couch

Let's start by articulating Christopher Bollas's thoughts on the couch, based on the assumption that, at a primal moment, the *self* and the object are experienced as being the "same thing". Bollas's reflection on our theme is certainly influenced by Pontalis's theorising on dreams. Pontalis writes:

> My hypothesis would be that every dream, as an object in analysis, refers to the maternal body ... Dreaming is, first and foremost, trying to maintain the impossible union with the mother, to preserve an undivided totality, to *move in a space prior to time* ... That's why certain patients implicitly ask us not to get too close to their dreams, not to touch or grind the body of the dream, not to disarticulate the "thing-presentation" into "word-presentation".[1]

The influence of Pontalis on Bollas, as well as being explicit in interviews, is notable when Bollas writes "when the Freudian aims to fragment the dream and examine it in parts, there is an objection. 'Leave mum and me alone!'"[2] Both authors believe that dreaming is a kind of return to the mother's body. However, we'll see that Bollas goes a little further to reflect on the couch. He states:

> The position Freud asked his patient to be in – lying on the couch – was a strange intermediate stage between the sleeping thinker and the waking thinker. It's a stage between life in the world of the mother (or what I called the maternal order) and life in the world of the father (or what I called the paternal order).[3]

Bollas is referring to the couch as a medium, an in-between space between two states. If we focus only on the first part of his remark, we might be led to think that Bollas is alluding to the hallucinatory mode of dreaming – the root of thought – but also to what is called "intentional" thought, with the intervention of conscious processes and crossed by the reality principle, if we are to speak in Freudian terms.

DOI: 10.4324/9781003681212-9

However, Bollas's theoretical thinking, in general, is more directly concerned with the intermediary space that exists (or doesn't exist) between the self and the other, as well as the different states and forms of functioning of the *self*. His theorising investigates, above all, the self-object relationship (internal and external), the relationships between internal and external spaces and the objects that make up and interrelate in these two spaces/worlds. Internal/external objects are not differentiated by the baby in their first object encounters (for example, with the mother, with the breast). The baby experiences an object stage in which the action of the mother-object is also experienced as its own. Prototypically, Bollas states that this encounter and relationship between mother-baby objects is what creates a transformational experience. From the point of view of an external observer of this scene, we could say that the baby experiences the relationship with the object-mother as a relationship with a transformational object. In relating to this object, the baby transforms itself incessantly. I will return to this idea, in other ways, later on.

If being on the couch means being between two psychic functions, as stated at the beginning, and if we accompany this phrase with our free associations, we can also read it as the "coexistence" of being an "individuated" self (paternal order) and being in a fused functioning with the other (being as a mother-self – maternal order). Analytical work on the couch takes place *in an* in-between space, oscillating between states. Dreaming – as a surrender to the mother's body (as Pontalis describes it), a fusion – would be something made possible by the couch, as we have already seen in Winnicott, while at the same time the couch would also mark separation, fostering the emergence and development of the self from that object-body. Therefore, I believe Bollas's theorization would lead us to understand the couch as a kind of other-object of support and holding, enabling a complex emerging from it. If the basis of Bollas's theory posits the transformational experience[4] as originary, and this derives from the relationship with the mother, the couch would be that prototype/replica of an object-body that fosters the analysand's self-development.

I believe that Bollas allows us to think about a base-couch that replicates a paradoxical functioning of an "in-between" character, of being mixed with the other-couch (mother's body) in the relationship (maternal prototype and often part of the transference as well) and, at the same time, being alone with oneself, with one's own body resting, with a "clear" visual field, with the possibility of evoking an internal and/or external construction of the past or the future. It would be through the evocation of transformational experiences already processed – of having been transformed by experiences, especially the earliest ones arising from the mother–infant relationship – that the desire and the space for new psychic transformations would open. For Bollas, the analytic situation invites regression:

> both participants regress together. The condition of the environment – one lying on the couch, the other sitting comfortably, free to look into the middle distance – the long periods of silence and the talking without waiting for

> a response: everything harks back to the first years of being. The difference, of course, is that, as both participants are now intellectually adults, there is a return to an earlier form of thinking equipped with more sophisticated unconscious capacities, as well as more developed forms consciousness.
>
> Both the patient and the analyst know that, however non-verbal the experience may seem, both will try to put into words retrospectively what they were thinking.[5]

Therefore, both members of the pair benefit from the use of the couch, as it helps them regress to previous stages of psychic functioning, including the non-verbal ones, which are also fundamental to the proper functioning of free association and floating attention. I'm quoting the author directly so that we don't lose the essence of his enunciation.

> Lying on the couch, with the physical sensation of being supported by this physical object; being physically close to the analyst and their person; the relief and pleasure (even in the midst of pain) of the analyst's apparently undivided attention to the self; the marvellously secure experience provided by the temporal dimensions ... [time and continuity of sessions]; the "cradle-like" experience one has of the objects within the analytic space when observing them, those eternally familiar objects that come from one's internal world; the intrinsic permission to let oneself fall into unconscious dream states of the self, simply allowing oneself to feel oneself, to encounter different experiences and to recount them to the analyst, when from time to time a discovery is made. Even when the issues are Oedipal, they may be like being held by the mother while talking to the father about being his child.[6]

In other words, we could say that the couch opens up to a radical experience. In it, all the manifestations of the *self* can coexist. There is dependence, the need for support, regression to primary functioning, and at the same time there is the mother, the father, the Oedipus, the conflict. Perhaps we can say that his conception of working on the couch is to live the conflict (paternal order), supported by the maternal order (*holding*). The couch becomes a cot (for genital sexuality and polymorphous sexuality) and helps to work on even the most aggressive oedipal impulses. It allows the *self* to manifest itself in its forms and stages.

The work on the couch is an "in-between" of the maternal and paternal orders. For Bollas, free association fluctuates "between the oneiric world of life within the maternal ambience and the lucid world of paternal laws and socialisation".[7] And, of course, as he makes clear in his work, the words "mother" and "father" represent functions, so they shouldn't be taken in their concreteness.

In fact, Bollas discusses the oscillation between states or the overlapping of states that encompass both the most primitive stages of the psyche and the most neurotic manifestations. Thus, even when he thinks about hysteria and sexuality, he doesn't give up thinking about the constitution of the *self* together.

In his book *Hysteria*,[8] he points out that the analysand "invests the couch, the silence, the corpuscular environment (two bodies breathing together) and eroticises the transference, which becomes an object of love".[9] He also states that hysteria is centrally characterized by the opposition between love and sexuality, "when one observes that the hysteric sees sexuality as a form of separation from maternal love".[10]

From this perspective, the use of the couch can be understood as an instrument that "fluctuates" its function between *evoking* the primary object and its character of care, and *evoking* sexuality (infantile and genital), according to the concept of *evocative object*, which will be presented later. The couch is an instrument that "floats" and superimposes various layers of the analysand's internal times and self-states. The body is always present, and "upon coming to a psychoanalysis, clothing her self in the couch, the hysteric re-(re)presents the body that needs to be seen and reinterpreted".[11]

Bollas's perspective emphasises the need to go into the parts of oneself that are failing to interconnect. "The psychoanalyst is therefore a father and mother combined, a figure who cures the hysteric, using the paternal symbolic function in order to evoke and transform the memory that the baby has of its mother," and this involves talking about everything that involves the body and sexuality. The pure, non-sexualised mother doesn't exist; her sexuality is there from the start, even if it isn't understood as such. The couch would serve both the expression of the *self* and the expression of sexuality at the same time, because the *self* and sexuality are not dissociated.

If we're talking about a couch invested with sexuality, it doesn't matter whether we're talking about the couch as the mother's or the father's body, depending on the analysand's sexual orientation and the state of his or her *self* that the analysand is presenting at a given moment – especially since Bollas refers to functions. However, it is important to point out that the couch-object serves as a receptacle for masturbatory,[12] oedipal and forbidden fantasies, as previously discussed in light of Ferenczi's contribution.[13]

When discussing regression to primal functioning,[14] Bollas goes on to elaborate his thoughts on the potential uses of the couch – though not before noting that some analysts seek to downplay the significance of the psychic and clinical phenomenon of regression:

> Some classical analysts object to the idea of facing and managing a regression because they sincerely believe that such a notion is ill-conceived and potentially dangerous. Other analysts protest because they believe that this point of view asks something of them that they cannot fulfil. This is the case for many analysts who have listened to case presentations where there are reports of success in managing regression to the object of addiction, because this realisation can force the painful recognition that a practice of analysis working with a different model of mind can have a successful outcome. It's

> hard to resist the temptation to invalidate a clinician of a different theoretical persuasion with a frequent remark such as: "that's not real analysis".[15]

In his view, profound questions arise: What is psychoanalysis? Is there such a thing as "true" psychoanalysis? If so, would that mean there are also "untrue" psychoanalyses? His theorising has consistently sought to avoid totalitarianism,[16] to emphasise the importance of singularities and theoretical differences as enriching the psychoanalytic theoretical-clinical frame. Regarding regression (as it occurs on the couch), Bollas cautions that the analyst should pay attention not only to long-term regressions, but also to periods that can be brief – even several short periods within the same session. "The core of the regression to dependence in psychoanalysis is a common abandonment on the part of the analysand of reporting or thinking about; during the silence, he experiences something else."[17] Bollas describes that the analysand starts to use a receptive capacity in which, "within himself", the analysand starts to relate objectively. There is a mental process of evocation, so that the deepest part of oneself begins to emerge. It's important that we follow his comments on the psychic processes during the regression process in detail:

> **1** After an important period of analytical work, or after the pleasure of the anticipation of an analytical session, or after a period of talking, the patient becomes oblivious to the presence of the analyst as interpreter. **2** The patient is in a kind of "twilight state" in which they find pleasure in lying on the couch, listening to the sounds of the analytical world (such as passing cars, the ticking of a clock or the sound of voices). He finds pleasure in the analyst's presence, the sounds of his stomach, his breathing and so on, which are felt to be comforting and continental. **3** After concentrating on the physical sensation of pleasure in being held by the couch and the acoustic sensations of hearing the sounds of the world, the patient falls into a state in which thought processes appear benignly "white". Thoughts arise in response to sensory stimuli, such as sounds or objects visible in the consulting room. Patients report that they often look at one of the objects in the room, but see it in a blurred way, not in order to interpret the object, but simply to get lost "inside" it. **4** There is a subtle transition from hearing, seeing and feeling the properties of the outside world to hearing, seeing and feeling the inside world. There can be a continuous interaction between the two worlds. Winnicott calls this the intermediate area of experience. However, this transition is not thought to be fundamentally pleasurable. **5** The patient reports being in the midst of discovering something important and new. I believe this is a shift from reception to evocation. It is from within this internal state that a dream can suddenly be evoked or a memory can emerge. Even so, the desire in such a state is not to narrate. The dream or memory evoked is part of the arrival of a condition of the self that is being

> evoked. In many times, the patient will report that during this state they saw themselves inhabiting an image, such as a chest of drawers in a playroom, a garden, a picture book, a car. "Seeing" these objects doesn't inspire meaning, but seems intrinsically pleasurable and meaningful. There doesn't seem to be any urgent need to understand this position. **6** This state may not be reached, as the person can only get to the above stage before leaving it to report the dream or work out something important with the analyst. However, occasionally the evocation of images (as opposed to thoughts, words or abstractions) inspires some deep affective state. The patient may feel deeply moved as a result of this imagining. This in itself seems to further deepen the ego's capacity for receptive evocation. **7** It is after the stage of imagining and feeling (probably what Masud Khan means by the experience of being) that a person regressing into addiction can suddenly "see" the meaning of everything. I find that exceptionally difficult to describe. I believe that what happens is almost a metonymic act. The image is part of the self-object experience and the affect deepens the memory. At that moment, a patient can suddenly discover something about their mother, their father or himself. Something they had never thought of before, but which was part of the unthought known. Some patients may burst into tears. Others behave as if they have experienced a revelation. It is very important that the analyst remains silent and deals with the situation without acting on their curiosity. Throughout much of the process described above, there is a need to experience this discovery in privacy, as the person may feel that they must preserve the privacy of their experience before reporting it to the analyst. There may be a fear that telling the discovery is tantamount to losing it. **8** Finally, there is an intense need to tell the analyst. I've never found the experience to be accompanied by a fear that the analyst won't be able to understand it. It's as if the patient believes (perhaps necessarily) that the analyst has been part of the experience from the beginning and depends on the analyst's ability to provide this. There is great joy in the discovery, even intense pain, and the patient may need to talk to the analyst at length.[18]

We can see that, for Bollas, the couch can also be a kind of protective and acoustic shell, like a warm lap or a mother's womb, echoing a mixture of internal and external sensations in a continental way and with a potential for revisiting contact with oneself and, at the same time, with a transformational potential. "A patient can change from a sensation on the couch to a perception of internal states of their body. They can change from listening to the sounds in the room to hearing a musical chord that passes through their thoughts, or they can remember the sound of someone's voice."[19] The analyst's patience and respect for the analysand's silence and time in this process seem to coincide with Ogden's thoughts on the need for privacy. His description of "benignly empty thought processes" is also interesting: the mental images that occur to him during the process don't inspire him with any meaning first. It's only "after the stage of imagining and feeling that a person in regression to dependence can suddenly 'see' what it's all about",[20] as if all the sensory and imagery experiences evoked in those moments, are part of a person's self-object experiences and are part of the "unthought known" that lives within that person. As Bollas points out, it is difficult to explain in words everything that is at stake in regression; and, if there is no "explanation", perhaps it would be better not to saturate it with comments, leaving the reader to re-read Bollas's quote (taking it as a theoretical object of use) and to be able to relate closely to his proposal.

The transformational potential of object relations is craved by the *self*. For Bollas, we are always relating to and using all kinds of objects, especially for transformational purposes. We want encounters with objects to bring us something new and/or evoke transformational processes in us. If Freud says that the psyche yearns to satisfy the drive, Bollas would be saying that the *self* seeks the transformational aesthetic experience from (in favour of developing the potentials of) object relations. The author proposes that we think about "evocative objects":

> as we wander through our worlds, we come across objects, whether natural or man-made, whether material or mental. For the unconscious, there is no difference between a material and a non-material evocative object; both are equally capable of subjecting the *self* to a complex inner experience.[21]

Bollas is dealing with objects that are already internal, or from the external world – or the relationship between the two – that evoke not only memories and experiences, but also states of transformational functioning that include processes of previous self-object transformations. In his conception of the psyche, there are procedural registers and not just representational ones that can be evoked through objects present in "our worlds", including inanimate objects from the external world. The consulting room and the couch serve, above all, as evocative objects[22] that evoke both the oneiric and *reverie* function and the body-support-mother function that serves to transform and complexify the psyche through experience. They evoke sexuality, oneiric functioning, Oedipal issues, the traumatic and/or what needs to come from each analysand. "When used by the *self*, [the objects] may – or may not – throw the individual into a complex psychosomatic experience."[23]

Therefore, although Bollas follows Winnicott's lead in understanding/listening to the couch as a corporeal object, he adds important reflections, especially the idea that the couch-object serves as a *medium* of evoking records of internal procedural functioning that need to come to the surface, either as a function of working-through the traumatic, or the very emergence of creativity. I realise that Bollas wants to elucidate how a regression would lead to the maximum stage of self-creation – the great creative moment, the core of the creative process, from which all the others derive. The analysand's need to enter this stage would be to "seek" the creative and transformative act. This hypothesis can be further developed in the second part of this book. Here we are interested in following Bollas's reflection and understanding that evocative objects transcend what we are thinking about the use of the couch, and their function applies to all the objects that make up the consulting room. In his book *Forces of Destiny: Psychoanalysis and Human Language*,[24] Bollas emphasises the importance of the aesthetic elements that make up the reception room or even what is outside the window:

> Whilst sitting in my chair, outside the patient's field of vision, I look differently at the various objects in my visual field. Could it be that the analyst's visual experience of their object world is unconsciously coordinated with the patient's discourse and the analyst's transferential use of it? I often look at a beautiful, long, not entirely white wall opposite me. During the course of the day, the wall registers light in subtle ways, which is emphasised by the fact that its surface is uneven, allowing the average intensity of the light to vary. I contemplate the wall, often attracted by the figurations of light, or else analysing it as a concrete eternity, as different patients pass by, at different times, and, I'm sure, for different reasons. Although I have paintings, ceramics, oriental rugs and other objects in my visual field, I'm sure that some of my interpretations have been, to coin a phrase, "inspired by the wall".
>
> I observed a schizophrenic woman during her analysis. She spoke rarely, and after a long time working with her, when the fabric of coherent thought began to weaken and I felt somewhat lost, I was aware that while I was listening to her, I was always looking at the different patterns of light on the wall, or at the cloud formations I saw through the window, but I never "travelled" around the room looking at "internal" objects …

This quote is relevant because it alludes to other inanimate objects[25] in the consulting room – other than the couch – and even includes the external view from the consulting room, the clouds, the wall and its "white screen", as auxiliary objects in the analytic process. Bollas refers to some elements that would be in the analysand's field of vision and others that would be in the analyst's – or shared by both – making some questions about the elements that make up a *setting* more complex. After all, Bollas points out that all the elements available in the field of vision influence the listening and speaking of the analysand and analyst – a point that could also be taken into account in the discussion about face-to-face analyses.

Implicitly, I believe that Bollas is responding to the fact that avoiding meeting eye-to-eye doesn't mean leaving the analysand with a blank stare. There are other objects, elements that can help with transformational experiences in analysis. We always have countless objects that can evoke transformational experiences.[26] Regarding the "cloud formations" evoked by Bollas in the selected quotation, I declare that these will serve as an essential metaphor to be explored in greater depth in Part II of the book, based on the theoretical frame developed therein.

In the last quote, it is also important to note that there is mention of a schizophrenic woman in analysis. In his book dedicated to schizophrenia,[27] Bollas summarised the first 20 years of his practice by saying that he treated some psychoneurotics, but most of his treatment involved "severe disorders", such as manic-depression, psychotic hysteria, paranoid disorders, psychotics in general. He attended on the couch, and his clinical vignettes illustrate the point.[28] His work includes clinical passages that elucidate quieter periods of regression. Even in material with a "crazier" content, however, the technical handling resembles (or is perhaps no different from) interventions that Bollas could also have made with neurotic analysands, since he proposes to work with the regression of any analysand and therefore does not strive to conceptually establish any technical differentiation in this sense.[29] On the subject of analysing psychotics and the possibility of them lying down on the couch, he poses quite a question for us to think about.

In a book dedicated to schizophrenia, Bollas states that it is true that many schizophrenics who are heavily medicated, hospitalised for a long period and left without anyone to talk to can regress in their ways of thinking, speaking and behaving, fitting into a conventional stereotype of a person who cannot mentalise or make use of a symbolic order. However, he says it is necessary to separate the causes of this deterioration. Bollas questions whether the causes of these serious deteriorations are intrinsic and characteristic of schizophrenia, or whether they are, unfortunately, more often true for the schizophrenic who is abandoned – left in a degraded state that results in psychic withdrawals that compromise mental function.[30] From this perspective, his position is that the "loose associations" of these patients cannot be neglected or thought of as not worthy of analysis.

Notes

1 Pontalis, 2005.
2 Bollas, (2007a) 2013a, p. 8.
3 Bollas, 2007b, p. 9.
4 Let's refer to the explanation of the transformational experience in Part I, Chapter 5, "André Green's couch – the dream model, other contributions and misreadings", p. 29.
5 Bollas, 2009b, p. 15.
6 Bollas, (1987a) 2018a, pp. 174–175.
7 Bollas, 2007a, pp. 9–10.
8 Bollas, 2000a.
9 Bollas, 2000b, p. 38.
10 Bollas, 2000a, p. 40.

11 Bollas, 2000a, p. 62.
12 For example, Bollas's analysand wanted to lie on his stomach to experience the sensation of rubbing his penis against the couch. In this case, the couch represented and evoked the incestuous and conflictual nature of infantile sexuality (Bollas, 2000b, p. 193).
13 See Part I, Chapter 2, "The couch, the child who lives in the adult, and the technical daring of Sándor Ferenczi".
14 Bollas, (1987b) 2018a, pp. 173–186.
15 Bollas, (1987a) 2018a, p. 174.
16 Krüger, 2021, pp. 31–40.
17 Bollas, (1987b) 2018a, p. 175.
18 Bollas, (1987a) 2018a, pp. 175–177.
19 Bollas, (1987b) 2018a, p. 178.
20 Bollas, (1987a) 2018a, p. 178.
21 Bollas, 2009, p. 50.
22 According to Peter Gay, Freud's numerous antique books and works of art delighted his analysands. I invite the reader to return to Part I, Chapter 1, "Sigmund Freud's couch-reminiscence", to think of the inanimate objects offered by the analyst in his consulting room as intrinsically linked to how each psychoanalyst views psychoanalytic practice. In Freud's case, his fondness for archaeology is linked to the idea of treating "reminiscences" of other times. From this point of view, his objects of ancient art would therefore be a materialisation that would evoke "reminiscences of other times" in the analysis room itself (Gay, 1989, p. 168).
23 Bollas, 2009, p. 50.
24 Bollas, (1989) 1992, p. 72.
25 As we'll see in Part I, Chapter 14, "Other authors and different approaches to psychoanalytic work from the couch", Richard Waugaman is concerned with demonstrating transferences directed towards inanimate objects in the analysis room, especially the couch, and reporting on various clinical situations.
26 Bollas is the author of *the* essay *Architecture and the Unconscious*, in the book *The Evocative Object World* (2009a), about cities and their architecture, theorising his experiential proposal through evocative objects beyond the *setting*.
27 Bollas, 2015.
28 In addition to the clinical cases in Bollas (2015), Bollas mentions the couch in serious cases in *Three Characters: Narcissist, Borderline, Manic Depressive* (2021), as well as situations involving breakdown in *Catch Them Before They Fall: The Psychoanalysis of Breakdown* (2013).
29 As we will see in Part I, Chapter 14, "Other authors and different approaches to psychoanalytic work from the couch", Danielle Quinodoz follows a similar perspective. Her interventions are designed to talk with both the more neurotic and the more psychotic parts of her analysands at the same time.
30 Bollas, 2015, p. 66.

Chapter 8

A distant couch in Jacques Lacan?

Even though we don't find many statements by Lacan that discuss the status of the couch, it is important to try to evoke its role in his clinical practice, given the author's importance to the psychoanalytic community. It is necessary to begin this chapter by warning that it is partly Lacan's reflections, but that it also draws on some contributions from other authors. The chapter is based on comments from theoreticians and analysands, even more than on Lacan's sparse words about the couch, although there are a few passages to comment on. After hesitating over whether or not to include this chapter in the book, I decided to keep it more for what it can continue to foster in our discussion than to try to achieve some supposed fidelity to the author's thinking. My focus is to reflect on ways of using the couch, and everything that follows is valuable in this regard.

The couch was not the subject of further discussion by Lacan, but in 1976, in a short passage, it is mentioned as a type of bed – and compared to a hospital bed[1] – alluding to a place where the symptomatic rests. Earlier, in 1955, he mentioned the "longitudinal axis of the couch",[2] at one end of which is the figure of the analyst, signalling that psychoanalysis is a "science of mirages", due to the alienations it brings to light, even though its purpose is to "hide". His metaphor is interesting, since analysis is about confronting these mirages. "The subject is not face to face with the analyst. Everything is done so that everything is erased."[3] The couch, the not-looking, would help to dismantle these mirages, allowing the analysand, through speech, to bring out their cloudy visions in order to clear them up.

In a supervised case report, Lacan presents the summary of two dreams of an analysand. In one of them, there is a dream about a baby, which Lacan identifies as being the subject himself, and in the next, the associative line parallels – according to Lacan – the sea, the couch, the upholstery of the analyst's car and the mother, as well as date inscriptions that refer to the birth of the subject. Lacan seems to understand that this analysand is rather "preoccupied with a child about to be born" and that, in this case, his dream and his anguish would indicate the emergence of the subject itself.[4] Is this, then, an auxiliary couch-vehicle for the emergence of the subject (as an effect of the signifying chain)?

DOI: 10.4324/9781003681212-10

Lacan would probably refuse to think of the couch as a maternal-body-cloaked vehicle, emphasising a corporeal dimension, because a corporeal conception of the couch would mean, for him, emphasising the imaginary dimension and not the symbolic one. However, the associative line exposed in his clinical example leaves room for another psychoanalyst, supported by other theoretical-clinical bases, to understand the material and work with it clinically from another angle. After presenting a possible corporeal use of the couch in Winnicott and noting similar and complementary thinking in Anzieu, Ogden and Bollas, a report by Pontalis about his analysis with Lacan brings a new element: the distance between bodies. In an interview,[5] Pontalis said:

> He had a very particular position, he didn't sit behind the couch as usual, he slipped into an armchair in the corner of the small room and this armchair, in turn, was hidden by another armchair. He was truly in his own corner. There were two or three metres separating his corner from the couch, which was in the other corner. This change to the usual setup may not seem important, but with hindsight it seems to me that it was a new way of creating a certain distance between him and his analysand, of not being too close, not being glued to the couch. Some English analysts placed their armchairs practically on the couch, a few centimetres away, breathing the same air, sensing each other's breath. With Lacan there was distance.

From this perspective, Winnicott would certainly be one of the Englishmen who would be close to the couch, "perceiving the breath of each person". Pontalis's account aims to highlight a radical difference in the function of the couch based on a notion of distance, whether thought of by Lacan or not. Winnicott favours the rhythm of the breath and, by placing himself close to the couch, he would be affectively and bodily available, while Lacan would be distant. Preserving one's space? Preserving the analysand's space? Is there any conscious intention in this supposed distance? Would more absence lead to more emergence of the analysand's word? The more the subject enunciates?

In this interview, Pontalis speaks of his experience of analysis as frustrating and criticises Lacan numerous times, the vast majority of which are related to an excessive use of power. Didier Anzieu made similar comments, adding new details such as Lacan's inability to deal with negative transference. His criticisms were even harsher, verging on a denial of ethics.[6]

Jorge Forbes[7] reports that, at times, while in session, Lacan would read the newspaper and also "leave the door open while seeing a patient; or even bring one analysand into the room while another was lying on the couch", which contributed to his poor reputation. To focus on Pontalis's criticisms, it's remarkable how he accuses Lacan of only worrying about whether his analysands attended his seminars, since they were in fact called by Lacan not analysands, but students. Throughout his interview, Pontalis speaks of his analysis in a tone of disappointment, leading us to assume that his perception of a "distance" may also be linked to this. It is impossible to measure whether this idea of distance from the couch was something Lacan technically thought up or not, whether he intended these effects or not. What is clear is Pontalis's dissatisfaction with this analysis; and his comment about the couch is, at the very least, food for thought – without forgetting that any analysis involves transference. After all, we can never take an account of what happened in an analysis as an indisputable fact and/or one that isn't permeated by the transferential relationship.

The Baranger couple[8] reflect on the distance between the couch and the analyst in a similar way to Pontalis, stating that an analysis doesn't run in the same way if the couch is close to the analyst or at a greater distance. In addition, they argue that the choices of physical space reveal the analysts' internal attitudes towards their analysands. From this point of view, it could be questioned whether there is a certain intentionality, even if only unconscious, for a supposed physical distance of the analysand from Lacan. If this hypothesis were realised, would there be a theoretical-clinical thought that supports a necessary "distancing"? Should the analyst adopt a position of closeness or distance from the analysand on the couch? Why and for what purpose? This depends on the theoretical vertex (perspective) from which the analyst is listening.

Lacan once spoke of the couch – in French, *divan* – as the *dire-vain*, that is, the path of vain speech that the subject takes in the free association established by analysis and that gives access to unconscious knowledge. The couch is the liberation of speech from the inhibiting power of the gaze, giving the voice a unique prevalence in the analytic experience. Lacan concludes that one does not speak in the same way in the sitting position as in the lying position, and it is in the lying position that one speaks of things relating to love. Lacan also drew attention to the importance of the voice object, emphasising that the drive linked to this object, the invoking drive, "is the closest to the experience of the unconscious".[9]

Once again, proposing a free interpretation (a free association) that does not pretend to be faithful to Lacan's thinking, based on this passage by Marco Antonio Coutinho Jorge, it is possible to see the couch as a *medium* that facilitates the word and also a *medium* that facilitates access to the field of sexuality and affections, since it is "lying down that one speaks of things relating to love".[10] If we go further and follow what has been articulated from the previous chapters, it would be possible to interpret the couch as a kind of embodiment of free association in the couch object/furniture, a materialisation of the internal movements occurring through the couch as a *medium*.

The "saying-vain" (not so vain) of free association would be closely linked to lying down on the couch, although in the terms *couch* and *dire-vain* mentioned there can also be seen as a somewhat forced analogy.[11] However, note that this theoretical construction is more mine than Lacan's or Coutinho Jorge's, as it would probably be more faithful to Lacan to think of the use of the couch from the point of view of the impossibility of seeing the analyst, who occupies the function of a missing object (as he is outside the analysand's field of vision).

In the previous quote, the attention drawn to the voice object and, of course, to the inhibition of the gaze is noteworthy, something that Antonio Quinet also emphasises.[12] Even supposing that Lacan doesn't see the thought put forward here as congruent with his theory, I suggest that we continue to seek our own interpretation and the possibility of asking ourselves if the couch couldn't also aid a certain connection with the corporeal dimension, by thinking that the form of speech is not the same in different bodily positions (sitting or lying down).[13] This idea opens up the possibility of thinking about horizontality as something common between the dream (fulfilment of desire), the sexual act and even original experiences – since human life and its first loves also develop from a horizontal position (at first, the baby suckles, sleeps, lives horizontally, etc.).

If, for some authors, it's interesting to think of the couch as a body-object, it doesn't seem that we can say the same about Lacan. However, if we were to discuss it in corporeal-real-spatial terms, and take up the distance that Pontalis mentions, we would be talking about a more solitary corporeal-space, distant from the other object, separated by another armchair, perhaps alluding more to the lack of the object than the encounter and use of the object. From this point of view, the progress of the session and its content (or the analyst's listening) would be linked, for example, more to the theme of lack. However, this is not Lacan's official position, which could well be objected to, but rather a possible interpretation of some of the traces exposed here. This corporeal-spatial dimension of the analytic space would be different from the corporeal-spatial dimension of Winnicott's clinic, in which the relationship with the object-analyst and the use of this object are more directly included in the scene. In Lacan, there would be a concretely physical object distance, which, from Pontalis's perspective, would also be a concretely emotional distance. A distance that could lead to a rationalising-intellectualising analysis and that would be distant from the human-affective dimension, according to his critique. The point is that the regression Lacan[14] is interested in is not exactly the one that evokes the "re-presentation" of the "child of the analysand" in the session. He makes it clear to us that, even if this were to happen, the point for him would be to work with the return of signifiers, which, obviously, refer back to the primal experiences.

Let's continue reflecting on some of the clues from Lacanian theory picked up by Antonio Quinet, which have proved to be extremely important contributions to continuing to expand the ways in which the couch can be seen in psychoanalytic practice:

> For Lacan, there is only one true demand to start an analysis – that of getting rid of a symptom. Lacan's response to someone who asks for an

> analysis in order to get to know themselves better is clear: "I'll get rid of it". Lacan doesn't consider this "desire to know oneself better" as something that has the status of a demand that deserves a response ... What is at stake in these preliminary interviews is not whether the subject is "analysable," nor whether they have a strong or weak ego to withstand the hardships of the analytic process. Analysability is a function of the symptom, not of the subject. The analysability of the symptom is not an attribute or quality inherent to it, as if it were something that belonged to it in itself: it must be sought so that the analysis can begin, transforming the symptom from which the subject complains into an analytic symptom.[15]

Therefore, after preliminary interviews, the couch is only indicated once a demand for analysis has been verified, which depends on the symptomatic manifestation and, above all, on the analysand's discomfort with this symptom. In this understanding, the couch becomes an instrument of auxiliary use in analysis, since it facilitates the emergence and work on the symptomatic, and the consequent dismantling of the symptom. When you lie down on the couch, you erase the image of the other, of the analyst's *persona*. The couch is a "cut in the *eye-to-eye*, in this body of preliminary *between-views*".[16] Coutinho Jorge points out:

> The transition from sitting face to face with the analysand to lying down on the analytic couch is, as Lacan said to Betty Milan in her analysis, a conquest for the analysand: "You didn't go to the couch, you conquered the couch! From now on, it's yours."[...] The neurotic needs to conquer the emptiness – beyond the imaginary – that analysis will give him, by speaking without addressing another as a person, but to the Other who constituted him as a subject.[17]

It is necessary to demarcate an active position in order to analyse, an implication. And the idea of "conquering the couch" only shows that Lacan doesn't think of it as a possible body (or substitute for the body) of the mother, as other authors do. If conquering the couch were equivalent to conquering the mother, the psychoanalytic process would be heading down the wrong path ...

From a Lacanian perspective, Claudia Riolfi[18] argues:

> The couch is the bed you lie on to stop dreaming. An analysis takes precisely as long as it takes for a person to realise that they can't find their answers in someone else. Until he loses hope of finding the object of his satisfaction in the world, the analysand insists on interrogating his past to find out what that object is.

It's important to return, one last time, to Lacan's cold distance in his analyses, as accused by Pontalis, in order to contrast it with the view of Suzanne

Hommel, Lacan's former analysand. In the documentary *Rendez-vous chez Lacan*,[19] there is a short passage in which she reports that her treatment was carried out in the opposite way to that described by Pontalis.

Suzanne Hommel: I'm from Germany and I was born in 1938. So I lived through the war years with all the horrors, the anguish, the aftermath, the hunger, the lies. I always wanted to leave Germany because of that. And from the very beginning of the first sessions, I asked Lacan: "Can I cure myself of this suffering?" I had thought that I could get this pain out of me through analysis. No, there was a way of looking at myself that made me realise: "No. You'll have to do this all your life." One day, during a session, I told Lacan about a dream I'd had. I said: "I wake up every day at 5am", and added: "It was at 5am that the Gestapo came to look for the Jews in their homes." At that moment, Lacan rose like an arrow from his armchair, came towards me and gave me a very sweet caress on the cheek. I understood: "geste à peau", the gesture …

Interviewer: He turned the "Gestapo" into a "geste à peau".

Suzanne Hommel: In a loving gesture. A gesture extremely affectionate. And that surprise didn't lessen the pain, but it did something else. The proof now, 40 years later, is that I still remember that gesture, I still have it on my face. It's also a gesture … an appeal to humanity, something like that.[20]

Suzanne Hommel's speech shows us Lacan making an aesthetic gesture, an intervention in the analysand's body, which would lead us to think of Part I, Chapter 2, "The couch, the child who lives in the adult, and the technical daring of Sándor Ferenczi". It's a staging that unites body, word and scene repetition with an internal transformation. The Lacan who lives inside Pontalis is not the same as the one who lives in Hommel. If Lacan went to her "like an arrow", he could even be far away from the analysand's couch, since arrows, unlike swords, are long-distance weapons. The fact is that it's more interesting to live with conflicting views than to find a univocal, absolute and dogmatic position.[21]

Notes

1 Lacan, (1975–1976) 2007, p. 98.
2 Lacan, (1955) 1998, p. 408.
3 Lacan, (1955–1956) 1997, p. 275.
4 Lacan, (1954–1955) 1995, p. 59.
5 Interview with Pontalis (2008), available at: https://www.revistapercurso.com.br/index.php?apg=artigo_view&ida=40&ori=entrev#topo.

6 The denial of ethics mentioned would be that Lacan not only concealed from Anzieu that Anzieu's mother had been his analysand (the Aimée case), but also invited Anzieu to analyse with him, leaving out this information, and this would have taken Anzieu years to acknowledge (Segal, 2009, p. 18).
7 Forbes, 1999, p. 10.
8 Baranger, Baranger, (1961–1962) 1969.
9 Despite Marco Antonio Coutinho Jorge's interesting observation, there is no bibliographical mention of this passage by Lacan (Jorge, 2017, p. 86).
10 In this sense, I'm not taking into account that, for example, "sexual intercourse doesn't exist", but rather taking his words from another angle. I'm taking this snippet as a stimulus to continue thinking. I have to admit that I don't feel suited to or identified with such conceptions. The most immediate and profound thing I can bring to the discussion is to interpret these phrases in terms of how they resonate with me.
11 See Part II, Chapter 17, "Some considerations on the history and etymology of the word couch/divan".
12 Quinet, 2009.
13 Particularities about the posture and its implications are developed by James Grotstein (see Part I, Chapter 12, "James Grotstein's dramaturgical and neuropsychic couch") and by Felix Deutsch (see Part I, Chapter 14, "Other authors and different approaches to psychoanalytic work from the couch").
14 Lacan, (1958) 1998, pp. 623–624.
15 Quinet, 2009, p. 16
16 Quinet, 2009, p. 42.
17 Jorge, 2017, p. 170.
18 Riolfi, 2014.
19 *Encounter with Lacan* (2011), directed by Gérard Miller.
20 The transcription used here is the one prepared by Luciano Mattuella in the book *O corpo do analista (The Analyst's Body)* (Mattuella, 2020).
21 Certainly, a psychoanalytic colleague more closely identified with Lacanian theorization than I am would develop this chapter in a completely different way. It would indeed be very interesting if something were produced along those lines.

Chapter 9

René Roussillon's couch in latency

We can find various clinical reflections on the frame and the couch in René Roussillon's work,[1] in the most diverse psychoanalytic modalities, including those that don't include the traditional consulting room. It wouldn't do to go into all the intricacies of the author's clinical thinking here, but to pick out a few points that will help us move forward. I will focus here only on the couch and its use/non-use.

> The psychoanalytic situation, the "analysing" space, apparently actualises a situation that "symbolises symbolisation", as a device that contains a theory of symbolisation "in act", … a device that forces the psychic functioning during the session to find the path of a suitable perceptual and motor suspension to activate the production of representations which, through the effect of rules and frames, are coerced into transferring to the language apparatus. The couch-armchair device places absence, the perceptual illusion of absence, at the centre of the process that induces and provokes etc. Motricity and drive are thus invited to transform themselves and transfer their movement into an operation of imagetic thought, a mode of operation that places representations of "visual" things at the centre of the process. André Green related this movement to the basic process of dreaming. The thing-presentation thus obtained is then coerced by the rule to be transferred in turn to the language apparatus, to take language as its object.[2]

By thinking of the psyche from the point of view of a tendency to always actualise what has been experienced symbolically, Roussillon tells us that the couch-armchair device points to an "illusion of absence" that induces representational movement and places imagistic thinking at the centre of the analytical process. Psychoanalytic treatment is based on transposing this experience into words, making language an object of labour. However, in addition to ideal conditions of psychic functioning, Roussillon also intends to deal with situations in which the psychic apparatus "does not 'contain' sufficiently well the tensions and impulsive excitations that travel within the device"[3] and, on this basis, opens up to thinking about other modalities beyond the direct use of the couch.

DOI: 10.4324/9781003681212-11

In the wake of what André Green proposes with the analyst's internal frame as fundamental and invariable,[4] Roussillon proposes that we think about the *couch in latency*. The internal frame accompanies the analyst even in situations in which the external frame varies from the "classic" one, when the use of the couch is abandoned for some reason. However, Roussillon would be adding an extra detail and helping with the frames in which the analysand is not resting on the couch. In the text *Psychoanalytic Conversation: A Couch in Latency*,[5] published in 2005, Roussillon presents the concept-title as fundamental to his theoretical and clinical thinking. The book in question condenses a large part of the author's thinking on this subject and will therefore be taken as the basis for this chapter. Any subsequent quotation that does not contain a direct reference is because it comes from this specific text.

Roussillon presents the couch as a "foundational" device, in the sense of founding, situation-origin, and in the sense of the original that acts on the psyche, especially of the analyst. He argues that the analyst's internal disposition is more important in defining an analysis than the external devices used, and states that "The 'free adaptation' of the analysis and the analyst, of the 'analytic style', seems to me to be the *sine qua non* of the creativity necessary for analytic practice."

The analyst's internal disposition would be the invariant of clinical practice. For Roussillon, it must be supported, "embodied", materialised. The analyst's internal disposition must be "represented in the psychoanalytic frame", and this must symbolise "in thing, in act", which would serve as a symbol for the analyst and the analysand. "It is not enough for the device to symbolise the symbolisation for the analyst, it is also necessary for the device to symbolise the psychic elaboration for the analysand, and this according to their own capacities." Because of this, and because of face-to-face treatments – those characterised by play, work with drawings, and so on – as well as the so-called extramural psychoanalysis, he began to postulate the *couch in latency*. This concept means that, even if it is not directly used in a particular treatment, the couch remains latent (and therefore unconsciously present) in the analysis session – since even if it is not materially used, it is in a state of latency (at least in the analyst).

> Several factors contribute to this "putting into latency" of the fundamental device and/or the importance within the device of the mute presence of the couch, which embodies and symbolises it. The first is countertransference. The analyst has done their own analysis within the couch-armchair device, which they link to psychoanalytic work. They then underwent their training, particularly the training that includes supervised treatments using this device. In other words, the couch and what it symbolises, the lying position and the invitation to passivity and the vulnerability of the loosening of defences that it represents, the analyst withholding their gaze, absence from visual perception – all the significant elements of the psychoanalytic

> apparatus are "present" and in a certain way symbolically inseparable from what analysis is for them. And it's not because the analysand is not lying down during the session and the "couch" isn't formally occupied that these essential characteristics disappear from their psychic functioning. They are in latency, remaining present as a backdrop, as a second-plane object of their way of listening. The couch is, moreover, most of the time perceptively present, in the analyst's line of sight, and, even in silence, it remains an organiser. Analysts receive their patients not behind a desk, but in a space where a couch is present.

Roussillon goes on to explain that this is not the only way in which the couch is implicit in any treatment, even if it is not used directly. "Generally, the indication of face-to-face or side-by-side work is made in function of the dangers where difficulties are sensed when trying to engage an analysis within the fundamental device", and it would therefore be in a kind of counter-reference to the couch that such modalities would be evoked.

The perspective that Roussillon presents is extremely rich, because he tells us about an "occupation" of the couch space, even when there is no one lying on it. The couch is invested and is organising for the analyst. Roussillon's perspective is that there is always a "couch function" invested by the analyst, even in appointments where it is not materially occupied. "For an analyst, trained as such, the fundamental device [the couch] is always present even when it is not used." His additions lead us to the idea that **there is no analysis without a couch**, even if we don't have an analysand lying on it. The couch accompanies the analyst internally, it is by their side and, consequently, will always be available to the analysand's gaze. Looking for an example of this condition, above all in the analysands, and not in the analyst, Roussillon evokes his experience from some clinical cases – among them, those of analysts in re-analysis – who would ask to be listened to face-to-face. These analysands, even if they were face-to-face, would direct their gaze more to the couch than to the analyst, because – according to Roussillon – the couch would serve as a "support" for the analysand, even if they weren't resting on it.

In addition to those analysands who would take the couch as a support, Roussillon points out that there would be those who would prefer to carry out their analysis face-to-face motivated by some need to communicate visually, pre-verbally and gesturally, or even by the fear that the couch and the regression it proposes could lead them to feel vulnerable and subjected to a position of passivity – although Roussillon is wary of theorisations that defend face-to-face as a perceptual protection in the face of psychic disorganisation. For him, a form of analysis that doesn't use the couch materially would be valuable for the analysand to enunciate transferentially from their own body – to communicate what is pre-verbal, in a kind of associative chain parallel to that of spoken language. Because "where the problem of visual perception is generally emphasised, I personally prefer to emphasise the importance of the 'messages' that pass through the visual channel and the transferential addressing that they imply", without failing to note that bodily and pre-verbal languages can also be expressed when lying on the couch, while reiterating that such a system of communication may prove faulty in certain analyses, failing to reach its potential.

> The postures themselves are also "very revealing". They "tell" a subjective position, a posture of being, they tell the story of the position adopted by the self in front of the object, the story of its fears or arrogance, its challenges or submissions, but also the object's responses to these messages, they report the "conversations" between subject and object. Often, for example, the position adopted by analysands on the couch indicates something of their internal posture. Curled up on the couch, rigid and ready to jump, one foot already out, or conversely "off" and on which everything will slide, there but already absent, the posture conveys a state of being. There are the positions in which the subjects "speak loudly" to a crushed little child, or those that, conversely and whatever they say, "speak softly" and are servile, like those of a child willing to do anything to collect a little investment and love ... Here again, I'm not trying to prove that such facial expressions or postures necessarily carry the trace of early childhood experiences, which carry these traits, but to emphasise that early experiences also bring their specific contribution to their formation or maintenance. If a certain mimo-gestural-postural aspect of the word comes to reinvigorate it, certain gestures, certain facial expressions, certain postures can no longer be considered merely as useful additions to habitual communication. They become significant because the first experiences come to mingle with adult maintenance, and find a way of infiltrating the subject's present without being transferred to the verbal language apparatus.[6]

His analysands would often propose a *psychoanalytic conversation*, a play of contents and forms in which one transforms the content and form of the other person's enunciation. This *psychoanalytic conversation* could take place with the analysand lying on the couch or sitting in the armchair. For him, there are different ways of thinking about the use or non-use of the couch, and the way in which any device is used can be more closely linked to the analysand's structural psyche or to what it has to do with a current moment.

Without necessarily referring to the analysis of children, Roussillon points out that this conversation takes place along the lines of Winnicott's squiggle game;[7] through this play and the analyst's verbal or postural placement, the analysand would be helped to start or continue an associative path – as something that engages continuity.

> The squiggle game (or rather squiggle play, more logical in the author's own terminology) invented by Winnicott can, in this sense, be considered the

> general model of the human encounter, the form of its "materialisation", its scheme: a proposition, partially unformed or awaiting form, calls for a "response" which transforms and "interprets" the first proposition, a response to the response which, in turn, transforms or shapes the response etc. ... it is the prototype of intervention in clinical practice.[8]

For Roussillon, it is in the associative link between analyst and the analysand that this analytical work takes place. For him, "the associative process characterises psychic functioning itself, and not just psychic functioning during the session".[9] More than an object relationship, Roussillon is concerned with thinking about the relationship "*with* the object",[10] including in it the potential for its use, with the analyst and the elements that make up the setting being part of this range of objects available for some kind of use.

Roussillon's theorising about the use (and non-use) of the couch privileges, in a way, bodily expression and gestures. He is concerned with "listening" to the analysand's bodily and sensory language. This prism would follow in the footsteps of Winnicott, Anzieu, Ogden and Bollas, but at the same time it opens up space to think of the couch as a symbol of internal support. If we follow this line of reasoning, we could think of the couch as a kind of object-support, either from the evocation of the analyst's internal couch (which is evoked when they attend, because they are or have been an analysand), or from the analysand who is face-to-face but has their eyes on the couch as a support when they freely associate, or even, essentially, from the analysand lying on the couch using its support (physical and metaphorical) for their free associations. The dimension of the couch permeates the various constructions of the treatment space, at least implicitly. We could think that this internal couch that accompanies the analyst would also apply to the child analyst and the analysis of children, or even to the analyst who works outside the consulting room. In this conception, the couch is always present, even if it's inside the analyst.[11]

Roussillon explores the idea of *psychoanalytic conversation* in depth, including its collecting, grouping and organizing functions in relation to discourse and the psyche. *Conversation* could be more constant for some analysands, but it would also be fundamental in all analyses, even if in a more punctual way. In this clinical proposition, Roussillon relies above all on *Analysis Terminable and Interminable* (1937),[12] in which Freud states: "During treatment, our therapeutic work is constantly swinging back and forth, like a pendulum, between a fragment of analysis of the id and a fragment of analysis of the ego. In one case, we wish to make something from the id conscious; in the other, we want to correct something in the ego."[13] In this perspective, the analytic work should operate in a constant interchange of layers and modes of intervention, ensuring that the treatment and the way of thinking about the setting do not proceed linearly. Asked about the differentiation between psychoanalytic psychotherapy and psychoanalysis, Roussillon states:

> There may be people who consider them very different. In practice, I work in much the same way. The idea is that I create or propose a device that I think is best for that person, always in psychoanalytic work. If the couch brings up intolerance, I do it without a couch. I work three times a week, four times a week. If the couch is better, I can have people lying on the couch working once or twice a week. What matters to me is thinking about the best device for this patient to do their inner work. If it's in front of me, fine; if it's lying down, so be it. In any case, I'm convinced that working with four sessions a week is not the same as working with just one session a week. This is because the patient won't commit in the same way if we see them every day or once a week. There are many differences in the process, but I don't think it's interesting to talk about them. Another important point is that I think this would be like sending a meaningless message to society; saying that psychoanalysis is not a psychotherapy for treatment. Intellectual psychoanalysis for philosophy students is diminishing more and more. It's over. It no longer makes sense! People come to analysis because we treat them. That's what we have to offer. I find it rather *snobbish* to think that psychoanalysis is not psychotherapy. A snobbery that rests on a misunderstanding of Freud.[14]

If, as Roussillon states, psychoanalysis is a form of psychotherapy, a differentiation between psychoanalysis proper and psychoanalytic psychotherapy (as Green conceptualises it) and the debates surrounding the use of the couch that permeate these discussions would not be in line with his thinking. The couch accompanies him as a psychoanalyst, whether he uses it concretely or not, and he is a psychoanalyst and psychotherapist in all cases, because these positions are not antagonistic. Roussillon will gradually reaffirm that the frame (and the couch as an essential part of it) must: "embody elaboration and symbolisation, show it, invite it ... Everything in the device must be constructed and ordered for this use: to say symbolisation and its conditions in this clinical encounter in 'thing', to say it 'in fact', 'in act'."[15] At this point, for him, each change in the device implies different embodiments, since different types of symbolisation come into play.

This chapter could have ended at the previous paragraph, but it's important to record Roussillon's positions here – which won't be developed in detail so as not to stray too far from the topic of the couch, but which will, in a way, relate to the theoretical-clinical construction present in Part II of this book. Firstly: the device is a potential *condenser*[16] of transferential processes; it is a "cauldron" for transference processes. Secondly: Roussillon tells us of a need to *theatricalise*[17] "the different signs that seem to be associated" in session. My later thinking will be similar and allied to these proposals by Roussillon, and the idea of condensing functions will be further developed, as well as themes involving theatricality. It's worth pointing out that these terminologies used by Roussillon, being Freudian in their essence, serve as a further stimulus to elaborate my own thoughts, and perhaps even leave the reader to imagine theoretical constructions based on these brief statements. The uniqueness of each analyst's theoretical and clinical thinking, as well as the unique encounter with each analysand, creates a unique process of analysis. "The mind is complex, and each type of *setting* allows us to analyse some aspects of it, but not others."[18]

Notes

1 Some texts are not being cited directly, but I think it's important to point out: Roussillon, 2010, pp. 21–38; 2016, pp. 230–245; 2018, pp. 121–131; 2013, pp. 257–276.
2 Roussillon, 2008, p. 26.
3 Roussillon, 2008, p. 27.
4 See Part I, Chapter 5, "André Green's couch: The dream model, other contributions and misreadings".
5 I base this on the translation by Eline Batistella, available at (no page numbers): https://issuu.com/psicossomaticainstitutosedessapient/docs/a_conversacao_psicanalitica_por_r_roussillon.
6 Roussillon, 2008, p. 79.
7 Winnicott, (1964–1968) 1994, pp. 230–243.
8 Roussillon, 2019, p. 45.
9 Roussillon, 2019, p. 69.
10 Roussillon, 2011.
11 There is something about the dimension of the couch explored by Roussillon that we could relate to the etymology of the word couch, which we will see in the chapter dedicated to it.
12 Freud, (1937) 1996g.
13 Quote taken directly from Roussillon.
14 Excerpt from an interview with René Roussillon, conducted on 28 October 2009, by Maria do Carmo Meirelles Davids do Amaral and Michael Harald Achatz. Available at: reneroussillon.files.wordpress.com/2014/08/entrevista-com-rene-roussillon.pdf.
15 Roussillon, 2019, p. 133.
16 Roussillon, 2019, p. 129.
17 Roussillon, 2019, p. 157.
18 Roussillon, 2011, p. 220.

Chapter 10

The analyst's creative process and the couch for Melanie Klein

How can we not reflect at least a little on the role of the couch for Melanie Klein? The materials we have for this are more historiographical than officially published, but they show that Klein's creativity and vision are too important to be ignored. It is by seeking a better understanding of the creative process of fellow psychoanalysts that we can come up with new ideas and propositions to keep psychoanalysis alive.

Melanie Klein didn't write directly about the status of the couch, even though her work with children obviously involves rethinking it. Her writings on the treatment of adults do not contain any peculiarities that we can discuss in terms of its function, at least not in a different sense from what has been presented so far. The fact is that the development of her work of analysis with children is intrinsically linked to the couch and its function. When she began her work at the Psychoanalytische Poliklinik in Berlin in 1921, Melanie Klein offered the couch and the method of free association to children,[1] usually from the very first day, showing great interest in the children's dream world.

With the exception of a few excerpts from the text *The Technique of Analysis in the Latency Period*,[2] there are no other official publications by Klein describing her indication of the couch to children, nor her annoyance at their resistance to her indication. However, the book *Melanie Klein in Berlin: Her First Psychoanalyses of Children*,[3] written by Claudia Frank and the result of research into Klein's archives, sheds light on the beginnings of Klein's analytical practice and her technical "experiments".

Researching from unpublished articles, notes and clinical diaries, added to other manuscripts and the records of the Psychoanalytische Poliklinik in Berlin – where Klein worked before she began to see patients in her home, around mid-1922 – Claudia Frank finds here the central role that the use of the couch held in Klein's earliest steps as a child analyst. Even though today we might see this practice as misguided, it needs to be understood in context. Just as experiments with hypnosis led Freud to create the psychoanalytic method, the couch plays a historic role in the development of Klein's technique with children.

DOI: 10.4324/9781003681212-12

As Money-Kyrle points out,[4] Klein "always assumed that the analysis of the child should be conducted in exactly the same way as that of the adult – with the sole exception that the analysis of verbal association should be complemented by the analysis of play". What Claudia Frank's publication illuminates is how seriously Klein took the principle reported by Money-Kyrle at the beginning of her clinical practice. Seeking to differentiate herself from the flirtation between psychoanalysis and pedagogy that had been going on for the previous decade, her initial impetus soon distinguished her from that usually followed when dealing professionally with children, which, in one way or another, involved the pedagogical aspect.

Melanie Klein was looking for the "essence" of psychoanalysis through the use of the couch. Her initial instructions for children to use the couch also reflected her interest in listening to their dreams and their symbolism. Only gradually did Klein come to realise that children could not "manage" to be on the couch in the same way as adults, and so she began to listen not only to the words of these analysands, but also to the symbolism of their play, seeing it as analogous to the mechanisms present in dreams. Although some analysts, including Hermine Hug-Hellmuth and Freud himself, had already signalled that play was endowed with displacements and condensations of the psychic world, it was Melanie Klein who managed to articulate the child's play within the clinic and develop it as a listening and intervention technique. It was little by little that the couch lost its position as the main analytical tool in favour of toys (and to play, obviously). However, we could conjecture that it is precisely a certain attention to the materiality of objects as instruments for accessing the Unconscious that may have helped Klein to see the toy as a way of accessing and intervening at the unconscious level of the highest potency. I believe that considering the full potential of the couch-object as an instrument of clinical access to the unconscious was what made it easier for Klein to shift its function to other objects, such as toys, as objects onto which fantasy can be projected.

This appreciation of the function of the couch meant that she never questioned its role in analysing adults, or proposed anything different about it, even though both her technique for analysing children and how they related to the consulting room were revolutionary. Except for a rare excerpt (which will be commented on later), we won't find any publications that propose any kind of reflection on the use of the couch in analysing adults. On the other hand, we do find the couch as an object of use, being part of the play and the dramatising in her analyses with children.

There are countless publications in which Melanie Klein analyses cases of children, in which the couch is part of the play or dramatising. The interaction with and through the couch can be seen in the clinical vignettes in her publications.

When writing about the analysis of latents,[5] Klein reports that there was a desire for them to seek the couch to be used as in an adult analysis (for example, Kenneth and Werner), as well as cases in which she insisted that the couch be used (for example, with Egon). It is also clear from the unpublished notes on the Greta case, among others, that some of the analysands in Klein's published cases may have sought the couch because it was their first recommendation – since they were treated at the Psychoanalytische Poliklinik in Berlin.

In a rare passage that mentions the couch from the perspective of adult analysis, Klein reflects on resting silently on the couch, accompanied by the presence of the analyst:

> There are other silences that express contentment, the pleasure of being with the analyst, of lying quietly on the couch, and I think they should be accepted without being interrupted by an interpretation. This has often been confirmed for me, when the patient starts talking again, saying that it felt very good to lie there quietly, feeling in silent contact with the analyst, whom they had internalised.[6]

In this excerpt, in addition to what she has explicitly written, it is possible to interpret that the scene is also about the pleasure of the analysand feeling at one with the analyst while lying on the couch, even though they are apart, as well as her respectful acceptance of the analysand's moment.

Klein elucidates a connection without words and understands the situation as the sensation of pleasure that the analysand would feel when internalising the analyst (and who she is representing). In the text *Envy and Gratitude*,[7] she describes the moment when an analysand gets up from the couch and says he was "well fed" by the session – which Klein understands as the recovery of the good object in its primitive form, so that we can think of the couch as what Winnicott would call a *holding* place. The couch plays the role of bodily support, while the analyst's listening and speaking intervene to nourish him and help him work on the mother object (or any other object) within himself.

Certainly, this scene does not constitute the enunciation of a profound thought about the function of the couch, nor does my reading of the issue under Winnicott's paradigm. However, other analysts could certainly reflect on the phenomenon in another way, from other theoretical understandings than that of internalisation. It might even be interesting for the reader to reflect on this clinical description based on the contributions of the authors we have not yet presented.

It's also interesting to think about the path Klein took when she began her clinical practice of analysing children using the couch, only to later shift the function of the couch-object to the toy-object, from the perspective of what Roussillon would conceptualise as *the latent couch*.[8] In other words, although she didn't use the couch as the main auxiliary object in her analyses of children, its function remained within Melanie Klein, perhaps even as an evocative object (according to Bollas),[9] offered to her gaze during her analyses. From this perspective, the function of the couch would always be present in children's analyses, even when it is not used materially.

Notes

1 Frank, (1999) 2009, p. 6.
2 Klein, (1932) 1997, p. 78.
3 Original title of the book published in German in 1999: *Melanie Kleins erste Kinderanalysen: die Entdeckung des Kindes als Objekt sui generis von Heilen und Forschen* [Frank, (1999) 2009].
4 Money-Kyrle, 1996, p. 18.
5 Klein, (1932) 1997, p. 78.
6 Curiously, Klein' reflection is in a book dedicated to analysing Richard, but she contextualises that she is talking about the analysis of both adults and children at this point (Klein, 1994, p. 233).
7 Klein, (1957) 1991, p. 237.
8 See Part I, Chapter 9, "René Roussillon's couch in latency".
9 See Part I, Chapter 7, "Christopher Bollas and the evocative couch".

Chapter 11

Wilfred Bion's embryonic couch

Wilfred Bion is another psychoanalyst who does not explicitly theorise the function of the couch. His references to it are embryonic but scattered, yet they open possibilities worthy of consideration. The following remarks seek to highlight some of these possibilities. With the exception of a short extract from the posthumous book *Cogitations*,[1] and another from *Transformations*,[2] the material I will present comes from his seminars and collective supervisions, full of clinical situations by Bion and others.

In a seminar for the Tavistock Clinic in 1978, Bion asks himself, when trying to gather important clinical information: Why might an analysand lie on the edge of the couch, instead of resting comfortably in the centre?[3] Without giving us a direct answer, even apologising for his imprecision, he answers his own question in a few words, implying that the reasons for this analysand lying on the edge of the couch are related to his foetal life and all the "debris", traces of psychic life from different times, that had accumulated. In São Paulo,[4] in the same year, also during a seminar, although Bion commented that he didn't know very well how to handle such a case, the same question was presented through a clinical vignette.

> I remember one patient who spoke freely and easily; he said he had no dreams and no imagination. Month after month, he attended every session, never failed, never got ill, never caught a cold. When he lay down on the couch, he seemed to have some difficulty, which I didn't worry too much about, as it seemed to be simply a question of adjusting his clothes and his comfort. But after about three months I began to think it was very peculiar. He would always lie down in a rather strange position on the couch; he would lie down and then raise his head as if he was fighting off some kind of opposition and trying to see his feet. He did this three or four times. I had no idea what he was doing or even how to tell myself what this peculiar movement was.[5]
>
> [...] it occurred to me that his precise and exact position on the couch could be understood as if he were lying on the edge of a precipice. His

DOI: 10.4324/9781003681212-13

> posture began to seem of a catalectic order. In fact, the whole analysis began to seem like a compulsive ritual – the same time, the same behaviour, no deviation from that position. The more I saw him, the more I thought that these were not ordinary communications and that my own interpretations seemed to follow a pattern.[6]
>
> [...] he had to keep chasing this Self around what seemed to be various anatomical areas. Making it clear that Self was not within the boundaries of what I call the body. I had to extend my interpretations over an area that had different boundaries – in fact, it had no limits. To express it, I would have to borrow a term like "infinite".[7]

It is very likely that the analysand described at Tavistock – lying on the edge of the couch as if on a precipice – is the same patient later presented in São Paulo. This analysand would be living on the precipice of himself, without limits, about to fall. No edges, an "infinity". If, on the one hand, the foetal prototype is not to be taken as a literal historical fact, but rather as a way of thinking about what still needs to be born – what needs to come into being in order to develop – on the other hand, it clearly denotes a lack of boundaries: a non-unitary self, fragmented, without limits and cast into infinity. There is no differentiation between the self and the other. We are talking about a suffering of *self-corporeal* indifferentiation. Although Bion doesn't mention it, it's clear that the analysand's use of the couch helped Bion to listen to his suffering. Therefore, we can think of an intersection between what is pathological and what are parts of the *self* that have yet to be born. For Bion, it is as if the analysand is immersed in the depths of the "unconscious" (in his own words).

The aforementioned clinical situation made Bion remember an intervention by Klein (as his analyst), when she said to him: "you feel mutilated, castrated, as if you had emerged from the womb".[8] Although he didn't feel that Klein's intervention made sense to him as an analysand at that moment, he felt that it made perfect sense to this specific analysand. In Bion's view, in this case, it was as if there was a "dangerous experience in which the mother, or the mother's genitals, mutilated the baby". He says:

> Additional experience over the years has made me realise that this is also true for the many rebirths that can occur between the moment we are born – in the obstetric sense – and the moment we die. This includes the moment when we emerge from one state of mind into another.[9]

In other words, each new "birth" alludes to an "infinity" of forms. In this way, the couch (and working from it) could be seen as a womb-container for new forms, new births and rebirths of the *self*.

Regarding analysands who declare a preference for being face-to-face with the analyst rather than lying on the couch, Bion explains that they don't understand that the couch isn't there to show them how inferior they are, but because it would be better for them if they used it. According to him, an analysand seen face-to-face "will resort to wearing dark glasses, feel uncomfortable/constrained, or look for a way to avoid being recognised – physically or mentally".[10]

In a clinical vignette from supervision, we also see how a white wall in the consulting room can be shown as a screen for scenes, like those in a cinema, projecting the mental life of the analysand, as a kind of "pre-word" moment.[11] Taking into account precepts linked to the form of communication, Bion added "we have to be careful with the tone of voice, the inflection and so on. There is not only the difficulty of having to give an interpretation, but also how we give it, what musical accompaniment we give to the words",[12] also making clear the importance of connecting with the emotional experience, with intonation, and what would be at stake in each clinical case.

Luís Claudio Figueiredo, alluding to the function of the couch, writes: "It is worth remembering that Bion quotes, with complete agreement, Freud's letter to Lou Andreas-Salomé in which he advocated such 'artificial blindness' to achieve the state of mind necessary to refine listening when the psychoanalytic object is especially obscure."[13]

Although sexuality is not at the centre of Bion's theorisations, when the theme of the couch is on the scene, it becomes present. In *Cogitations*,[14] he refers to a clinical situation in which the analysand – when faced with the couch not properly organised, as it usually would be – became very anxious, leading Bion to interpret that the couch was representing the analysand's discomfort with his parents' sexual intercourse – a situation similar to that reported in the Los Angeles Seminars.[15] When referring to an "accumulation of perceptions" – a mental construction by the analyst – Bion comments on having made the following interpretation: "I think you're really feeling like a baby lying on the couch. And nobody knows what that means. But, of course, it means that your parents had sex."

Although we can understand his intervention as an intention to emphasise, perhaps, "that which came before – that which precedes", we can't overlook the importance given to the primary scene and sexuality in Bion's interventions, at least in terms of his listening in relation to the couch, even though these issues are not emphasised in his theory. In São Paulo, in 1973,[16] we will also find comments and interventions by Bion relating lying on the couch to parental coitus. At least in these vignettes, Bion's interventions seem to be concerned with highlighting the baby (who would live in the analysand) and its emotional capacity, while at the same time referring to sexuality and its incomprehension. It's not my role to discuss the form of Bion's interventions quoted here, above all because they are vignettes, but they seem to me not to be endowed with much sensitivity, appearing to be overly rationalising, without taking much account of the affective dimension of the words used. However, we can see that, in his interpretations, the author tends to consider a variety of experiences that a baby can go through (quite primitive aspects), while at the same time referring back to the breadth of sexuality. Perhaps, with a certain freedom of interpretation on my part, it is feasible to think that Bion was paradoxically "listening to the couch": on the one hand, the couch is the place of the baby (a cradle), at the same time as it is the place of coitus (the parents' bed), performing a kind of integration between what is primitive and what is genital.

Bion's analysand, José Américo Junqueira de Mattos, recounting parts of his analysis, comments on his difficulty in analysing (and communicating) in English, saying that this distressed him and made him feel deprived of his ability to communicate, because expressing himself in English meant that he had to learn everything all over again. When he told Bion that, because of these circumstances, he felt as if he had been put on a Procrustean couch, Bion replied:

> You feel it's not easy to adapt to America. You came from Brazil and left your family, your job and your friends behind. You also left your language, your food, your habits. This change, this sudden rupture makes you feel crippled and deprived, as if you had to learn everything all over again. Look at the price you're paying to learn. However, can there be knowledge and learning without pain? [...] There was a time when you didn't know how to speak either and you pointed to what you wanted. You had the desire and didn't know how to put it into words. We could say that now you're being born into a new world. Think this experience has a long history. It didn't start now. For you, it revives your birth, in which you may, like now, have felt crippled and deprived, or mutilated and castrated. The first Procrustean bed you experienced was at birth.[17]

All these germinal ideas that come from Bion's interventions, although certainly of interest, they do not seem to me as crucial as a short extract from his book *Transformations*:[18] "Two people are present: me and a patient ... While he lies on the couch, I sit and imagine that a cloud is beginning to form ..."[19]

> I imagine that a cloud begins to form in the same way that clouds can sometimes be seen above a "hot spot" on a summer's day. It seems to be above him. A similar cloud could be visible to him, but he would see it rising from me. These are clouds of probability.
>
> Then other clouds form: some of them are new clouds, some are formed from old clouds, clouds of probability that have become clouds possibility.[20]
>
> The tension that is an essential part of the model is perceptible, as are the clouds. The clouds have increased; clouds of possibility have become clouds of doubt. Clouds of certainty appear; clouds of depression, guilt, hope and fear. Each cloud has its own "hot spot", but the cloud, like its analogue in nature, can move away. I associate pressure with tension and clouds.[21]

Bion is introducing us to an idea in which "clouds" come from "hot spots"; in this case, let's understand them as the human beings themselves and their psyches present in the analytical session – especially the analysand. It would be up to the analyst to try to "capture" what these "clouds" that come from emotional experience might be. Bion is talking about a model of tension and pressure (and, in this sense, supported by Freud, according to Bion himself). He makes it clear that, despite the appeal to a "visual" image reference based on "clouds", we could think of this metaphor from an olfactory, auditory and tactile perspective, using the example of the dog and its ability to sniff – in other words, it's not just a question of "seeing" clouds coming from the analysand, but also "sniffing" them.

His metaphors about clouds are not taken to be a concept, but rather a way of explaining his algebraic models. Bion seeks to equate ways of listening to intervention from his grid. In his mathematical models, the "cloud" must be replaced by a kind of "point", within an equation that concerns theorising about the Grid, its gradients, its elements, its preconception, etc., and it would be impossible to enter this field without deviating from our subject, the couch. Furthermore, I have to admit that I don't identify with and find it difficult to conceive of the psychoanalytic clinic under such mathematically explained models, which would consequently prevent me from elucidating them properly. If you are interested in discussing Bion's work from this point of view, I recommend that you look for good commentators. It's up to me to emphasise the metaphorical work and the production of forms present in the author's thought.

In our proposal to try to provide ways of listening from the couch, the idea that the analysand is "offering clouds" is very important. It's up to us to listen to them and, obviously, look for ways to work with them. Thinking about the psychoanalytic session from the point of view of metaphors that make use of "clouds" is central to the second part of this book, even though the thinking developed there does not make direct use of Bion and starts from other conceptualisations. One point that we will see later, as a radical difference from Bion's conception, is that he seems to use cloud more to refer to what is obscure and therefore needs to be "clarified", cleared up. I imagine he's talking about the "British clouds", which mix with the smoke from the chimneys and get in the way of the sunlight. The quality of the "clouds", on the other hand, which I intend to take as a basic metaphor for the clinical work in Part II, while still retaining the idea of clouds that hide something behind them, is that of "clouds" that emphasise other particularities, somewhat more tropical and playful, if I may say so.

Notes

1 Bion, 2005.
2 Bion, (1965) 1991a.
3 Bion, (1978a) 2005, p. 44.
4 Bion, (1978b) 2018.
5 Bion, (1978c) 2018, p. 91.
6 Bion, (1978a) 2018, p. 92.

7 Bion, (1978b) 2018, p. 98.
8 Bion, (1978c) 2018, p. 93.
9 Bion, (1978a) 2018, pp. 93–94.
10 Bion, (1975) 1994, p. 35.
11 Bion, (1978b) 1994, pp. 171–172.
12 Bion, (1978c) 1994, p. 193.
13 Figueiredo, 2020, p. 75.
14 Bion, 2005, p. 9.
15 Bion, (1967) 2013, p. 18.
16 Bion, 2018.
17 Junqueira de Mattos, 2016, pp. 20–21.
18 Bion, (1965) 1991a.
19 Bion, (1965) 1991a, p. 117.
20 Bion, (1965) 1991a, p. 117.
21 Bion, (1965) 1991a, p. 117.

Chapter 12

James Grotstein's dramaturgical and neuropsychic couch

James S. Grotstein devoted himself to thinking about the use of the couch from several angles that complement what we have examined so far, particularly in his paper, *A Reassessment of the Couch in Psychoanalysis*,[1] and in his book, ... *But at the Same Time and on Another Level* ...,[2] which covers the content of the aforementioned text with some slight modifications and extensions.

Let's start by clarifying his way of indicating the couch to the analysands in order to understand his thinking. In a fictitious and demonstrative dialogue, which would take place after the evaluation period, Grotstein would tell the analysand:

> Now that we've agreed to your entry into analysis, I'd like to introduce you to how it's conducted. One of the procedures is the use of the couch. Do you have any ideas or feelings about its use? The justification for its use began with Freud and his discomfort at being observed while immersed in his thoughts about the patient. In addition, he thought that the patient would feel more comfortable lying down. He didn't recognise that in fact, he had discovered the right hemisphere, an "alternative brain that switches on when the other switches off" when someone lies down in the presence of another person without being able to observe them with their eyes. This data processing system is sensitive to emotions, fantasies, illusions and the like and is less concerned with logic or continuity than the other. I think you'll be able to understand this by yourself. However, you should know that it won't be a requirement if it sounds uncomfortable or unsettling. However, the very reasons why you might find it unpleasant would be important for us to understand.[3]

Certainly, this is a distinctive style that even evokes neurological issues and Freud's inner motivations. However, Grotstein's thinking is more complex than this prototype indication that he offers his readers. He comments that Freud didn't realise that, through the use of the couch, he "discovered the right

DOI: 10.4324/9781003681212-14

hemisphere of the brain",[4] and that when someone lies down and isn't making eye contact, they would be activating a "shift" in the functioning of their cerebral hemispheres – in terms of information processing – from the left to the right side (or vice versa, depending on whether we're talking about left-handed people), highlighting research with children that showed a big difference in alertness when sitting or lying down.

The combination of being rested (less alert) and a consequent "shift" from the most used hemisphere to the least used – when lying down without eye contact – would help the use of free association. In Grotstein's view, swapping the predominance of the left hemisphere (sitting), which is more linked to organisation and linearity, for the right hemisphere (lying down) and its characteristic of looser, more fluid and irregular functioning, would facilitate the search for objects and sources on which to "lean", consequently helping with "association" combined with fluctuating thought – in other words, this would help free association.

According to the author, when we lie down, the right hemisphere "speaks", especially through visual impressions, imagination, fantasy and illusion.

Beyond this neuropsychic conception, Grotstein argues that "The use of the couch dramatises, exaggerates, and allows the unconscious to select. It can be concluded from this that lying down facilitates a shift from the real world to imaginative, phantasmagorical and illusory worlds". His understanding, following Freudian metapsychology, is that "the discharging action of the drives must be prevented in order to allow a verbal transformation", with the couch being an aid in this process.

For him, the role of the couch is to facilitate "the emergence and sharpening of the dramatic aspects of a person's inner life so that they can be recognised",[5] opening up space to view psychoanalysis from a dramaturgical perspective, in which, in the session and in the transference, a play is staged.[6] On the one hand, it would be an improvised "play"; on the other, it would be previously "prepared" to be revealed in session – in the sense of the internal that compels it to be dramatised.

From this dramaturgical perspective, Grotstein reinforces the importance of the couch, arguing that the sitting position and the face-to-face would diminish the intensity and authenticity of the *performance of* this "play". He returns to Lacan to point out that, when lying down, the analysand is only apparently talking to the analyst, because, in reality, they are immersed in their inner depths, "participating in an act of discourse with themselves through the analyst as a channel". As well as listening to the person on the couch, we listen to the text of the associations coming from their Unconscious. In the same way, the analyst's interpretation, even if mediated by the analyst's ego, aims to talk to the analysand's Unconscious.

Grotstein also comments on the usual fears that analysands, not yet initiated on the couch, would feel, such as falling asleep, entering states of dissociation or feeling abandoned, indicating that these thoughts/feelings are already setting in motion the illusory mode intrinsic to the use of the couch. His conception reinforces the fact that the use of the couch does indeed evoke a certain character of "unreality".

Grotstein tells us about an analysand who, when lying on the couch, feels the analyst to be frightening, incredible, intimidating, but who, when facing him when it's time to leave, sees the analyst regain his "human size".[7] In Grotstein's view, the couch offers "unreality", an "illusory mode" and the possibility of a functioning analogous to dreaming. He seeks to reinforce the intrinsic aesthetic character of the psychoanalytic session and what its frame offers, because, for him, "one can then conceive that the analysand's unconscious creates, writes, directs, produces and presents an enigmatic scenario made up of free associations".[8]

For Grotstein, it would be no less important to think of the couch from the perspective of the maternal function, without neglecting its neuropsychic perspective:

> Lying down makes it easier to reach the electroencephalographic brain state known as the theta rhythm, which corresponds to what Bion (1959) called *reverie* – the state that characterises the receptivity of a breastfeeding mother and the receptive state of her baby during breastfeeding. This corresponds to a trance-like state of optimal receptivity to impulses from within and from the external world with a minimum of defensiveness. In this state of *reverie*, the mother's *alpha function*, which Bion (1992) called *alpha dream-work* in his previously unpublished personal diary, is actively functioning in an optimised way. It's important to realise that the Bion's oneiric term *alpha*, which can be thought of as daydreaming or, more precisely, the continuation of the dreaming process in waking life, offers a new dimension to psychoanalysis.[9]

In this way, the analyst receives the analysand's associations in a waking dream state – and the analysand receives, as an intervention, what has been "digested" by the analyst in their *reverie* state. Grotstein argues that, since Bion, psychoanalysis no longer deals only with the Unconscious, but also with the *Inter-* and *Intra-Unconscious*, emphasising spatiality as an aid to the transferential process and to analytical work.

> The geographical location of the analyst *behind* the patient allows this spatial relationship to be realised and actualised as a vital metaphor, in which the patient can imagine sitting on the analyst's lap (when dominated by the fantasy of the analyst as a nurturer) and as a persecutor and "stabbed in the back" (betrayed) when the negative transference is predominant.[10]

Reaching the wakeful dreaming state depends on the trust established as well as on the privacy between participants, making it crucial that no gaze invasion occurs during the session. Grotstein reminds us that, although the mother's gaze is vital for the infant's psychic constitution, "the loss of the option to look opens the channels inward for each participant".[11] It is by looking inward that what is known as "intuition" develops, he argues. Consequently, the privacy of the gaze afforded by the couch is of utmost importance, both for the analysand and for the analyst.

Among the remarks that contribute to the reflection on the use of the couch, Grotstein highlights the ritualistic and formal character that accompanies its use, reminding us that candidates for training as analysts often feel pressured to persuade their patients to adopt it, largely due to institutional requirements – which ultimately conflicts with the very idea of conducting a good analysis.

For Grotstein, hybrid situations, where the analysand alternates between lying down and sitting up, can become part of the work. He tells us about an analysand who talked about "concrete" things in her routine life while sitting on the couch for a certain period of time at the beginning of each session, only to lie down later on and "start" the analysis.

While Grotstein is open to trying to understand clinical modalities that deviate from the traditional, although he doesn't discuss the details, he recalls that there are analysts who use swivel armchairs in the analysis environment and that their use certainly brings peculiarities to the way of listening and intervening in the clinic. Ana Lúcia Monteiro Oliveira,[12] for example, considers the use of reclining, swivelling and rocking armchairs for the analysand. She comments that this type of armchair offers a transitional function uniting and separating, the possibility of rocking, turning on one's back, looking and not looking, "hiding" and "returning". Based on her clinical practice, the author points out that the resource of having one's back to the analyst, in the swivel chair, is usually accepted by her analysands who resist using the couch, perhaps even because they feel more in control of "swivelling" quickly and/or putting their feet on the floor if internally they feel it necessary. She points out that many of those who started out using the recliner migrated to the couch within a few months. Even though some of them tried hard to avoid it, either because of neurotic resistance or because they were afraid of reactivations of the traumatic emerging, they ended up opting for the couch during the process – which is a creative and interesting modality.

Regarding the ways in which the couch and its function can be used, Grotstein tells us not to distinguish its use based on the frequency of sessions or any differentiation between psychoanalytic psychotherapy or analysis. He cites, as an example, several analysands he treated on the couch once a week. In these sessions, deep transference neuroses were established, and the material from each session was continuously and unconsciously interconnected, "achieving significant results."[13]

When thinking about indicating the use of the couch from a psychopathological point of view, taking into account severe suffering, Grotstein points out that each case must be considered individually. He[14] also points out that borderlines, psychotics and those suffering from post-traumatic stress tend to require the analyst's concrete gaze, but its indication should be considered on a case-by-case basis, since many could benefit from lying on the couch.

Grotstein also reports cases of analysands[15] with schizoid tendencies who, when they were on the couch, felt alone, fragmented and lost, and who asked to move on to face-to-face. However, after this passage, the analysands themselves signalled that they felt this modality was more superficial and showed a desire to return to the couch to "go deeper". In his view, "The patient on the couch feels freer to recover their deepest feelings, to dive into them and ponder them."[16]

Among all the psychoanalysts presented here, Grotstein's reflections on the couch stand out as the only ones to address neurological issues without ever deviating from psychoanalytic precepts. While his theorisation ventures beyond the boundaries of strictly psychoanalytic models of the psyche, he employs them solely to enrich his creative psychoanalytic understanding, working at the intersection between Freudian and Bionian elaborations, and even incorporating Lacan into his propositions.

Notes

1 Grotstein, 1995, pp. 396–405.
2 Grotstein, 2009.
3 Grotstein, 1995, pp. 401–402.
4 Grotstein, 1995, p. 396.
5 Grotstein, 1995, p. 397.
6 I would emphasise that this point – of seeing the session as the staging of a play – will be dealt with in more depth in the second part of the book, from another perspective.
7 Grotstein, 1995, p. 398.
8 Grotstein, 2009, p. 9.
9 Grotstein, 1995, pp. 398–399.
10 Grotstein, 1995, p. 400.
11 Grotstein, 1995, p. 400.
12 Oliveira, 2020.
13 Grotstein, 2009, p. 19.
14 Grotstein, 2009, p. 69.
15 Grotstein, 2009, p. 18.
16 Grotstein, 2009, p. 398.

Chapter 13

The couch as an aid to a filmic script in John Munder Ross

As well as being a psychoanalyst, the American John Munder Ross worked as an actor and director, above all with the *Harvard Theatre* and the *Harvard Drama Club*. As we shall see, his thoughts on the psychoanalytic session and the use of the couch ended up bringing his experience in the field of art closer to psychoanalytic work.

Ross points to the couch as an instrument to help "relax" unconscious barriers and defences, in a similar way to what André Green[1] proposes with regard to the dream model. However, Ross's theorising adds some interesting facets for us to explore. Just as Grotstein seeks to understand the use of the couch in a non-psychoanalytic discipline (neurology), Ross references the use of the couch using cognitive psychologist George Klein[2] and his aphorism "posture is perception".

For Ross, lying on the couch brings into waking life the aspects that Freud theorised about dreams and, according to him, by recommending the systematic and frequent use of the couch, without the possibility of seeing the other, Freud would be introducing to both the analysand and the analyst the work of the former's imagination in a completely innovative way. The couch would provide an essential opening to psychic reality. Not being looked at allows the analyst to "look inward" and reach insights at deeper levels regarding what the analysand expresses.

In his "splendid isolation" behind the couch, the psychoanalyst would reach a new level of empathy for the analysand's suffering. "The analytic situation is implicitly designed to alter the consciousness of both participants in different but mutual ways, contributing to another level of expression and communication. More specifically, the patient's oneiric (or rather hypnagogic and hypnopompic) condition tends to make the preconscious conscious."[3] For Ross, the analyst's senses and imagination must feel what the patient feels, particularly the tension, pain and self-protective resistances they provoke.

> The couch confronts analysands with various paradoxical injunctions – contradictions that make the analytic encounter inherently conflictual. They

DOI: 10.4324/9781003681212-15

> must lie down alone in the presence of another. As Lewin (1955) and later Stein (1965) interpreted the state of consciousness induced by the analytic situation, analysands must both dream and "observe" – that is, "observe" the dream state they encounter. In such *reverie*, according to Lewin, the voice of the analyst, like the voice of the archetypal father in childhood, becomes "the alarm clock", reorienting patients to their surroundings and the need to try to communicate what is ultimately ineffable. Lying on their backs like the archetypal baby, they are moved to become pre-verbal even as they are urged to speak, to put into words their visual images and bodily sensations.[4]

Furthermore, "for Freud, transference is a metaphor … a form of *imaginary play*".[5] In our psychoanalytic work, we all "*play*" with the "material" coming from the analysand. Ross says that it is part of the analyst's job to "listen to the music" and the "choreography of meanings" of the material in the session, each in their own way, according to what Rosen[6] called *pre-conscious illuminations*. In order to understand Ross's original thinking in more detail, it is necessary to follow directly, from his own words, how he works the session from what could be called a "film script", as well as the function that the couch fulfils from this perspective.

Let's follow the selected vignettes:

> Let me get personal for a moment and reveal how I receive and process my patients' communications and associations from a way of listening and reflecting that I have developed over the last twenty years of psychoanalytic work. When reading plays, epics, novels, short stories, and even journalistic or historical accounts, my immediate tendency is to visualise and listen to what the words on a page portray and create dramatic scenes from the "script". Most of the time I watch and, like the actor I once was, participate in the action from the perspective of one or other of the characters involved. In the process, not only do I see what I imagine they see – I always think in visual images – but I also feel what they feel, in my mind's eye, speaking and acting as I imagine they do. One of my joys in this performance is the ability to "become else" for a while and then return to myself.
>
> I see myself doing the same with the patients I'm analysing …[7]
>
> When the analysands lie down on the couch, I practically lie down diagonally in my Stressless recliner next to them. I look at my analysands from time to time, but not constantly. This posture makes it easier for me to translate the images and sounds transposed in their words into film sets, mainly "filmed" from the patient's point of view, although occasionally from a broader point of view or, less frequently, from another character or object in the narrative.[8]
>
> Most of the time, I try to stick to the patient's narrative and remain encrypted in their psychic reality, as I did years ago when I was playing a

> role in a play. But now, in a more private and silent way, as the drama unfolds in my own altered state of consciousness.[9]
>
> When I come across a dissonance, when a patient's words and the apparent apprehension of the moment don't fit into the "film" that he or she has conjured up in my mind, I find myself waking up from this reverie. It's at this point, faced with a rupture or distortion in the "text", with a contradiction and, consequently, a conflict, that I find myself experiencing a flash of anxiety or some other affective disturbance. After a pause, my floating attention narrows into concentration. It's at these junctures that I begin to prepare myself to intervene, to point out inconsistencies in the story.
>
> Away from the analysand's gaze, I feel freer not to respond immediately, not to speak until I want to. So, while I prepare to make what will be an interpretation of the defences, I can hold back and wait, making sure that the contradictions and affections that accompany them, as well as the manoeuvres employed to cover them up, are the patient's own.
>
> Having used myself, I try not to impose my ideas, expectations, prejudices and predilections on my patients, even when they want them. It's our job to challenge, rather than take at face value, the authority attributed to the analyst. And, once again, I reiterate that the couch facilitates this dimension of the process, safeguarding the autonomy of my analysands. When they enter the consulting room, the world inside, I hope, belongs to them.[10]

Ross's words are more precise than any comment that could be made, so I suggest we avoid being redundant. Perhaps it would be interesting to draw attention to the way in which he describes his imaginary process of listening, and I wonder: Don't we all imagine, in our own way, the scenes reported by analysands? In my listening, it has always been very natural to imagine the "characters" and "plots" offered by their communications. In this sense, Ross's merit lies essentially in proposing these "visualisations" of the analyst as a listening model in their own right. Nevertheless, it is no less important to emphasise the singular way in which he would work from the analyst's *reverie* and how this way of approaching the session reverberates in the analyst's mode of intervention.

The fact is that his thinking can resonate with other models of listening. The way Ross thinks about the couch is intrinsically linked to his way of listening and intervening. We could say that he is close to Thomas Ogden's theorising[11] about the need for privacy (based on not looking concretely) in the analytic pair. Thinking of the consulting room and the "world" within it as a "world" that belongs to the analysand could also be seen as something close to Christopher Bollas's[12] theorisation of the transformational and evocative object. Clearly, Ross's proposal to listen to the "dramatisation" of the material communicated by the analysand resembles Grotstein's[13] observations. We might, of course, continue to trace further parallels here, but the analyst-reader's inner work can also reach them in his or her own singular way.

Ross's theorising and his emphasis on the use of imagination (of analyst and analysand), as well as his way of thinking about the "roles" and "plot" present in the analysand's communication, become aids in listening and intervention. This comes close to what I will present in the second part of the book, making this chapter, in a way, a kind of introduction to what will follow. The complex simplicity that is present in Ross's way of enunciating his listening process means that his contribution can reverberate and continue to be rethought by the psychoanalytic reader.

Notes

1 See Part I, Chapter 5, "André Green's couch: The dream model, other contributions and misreadings".
2 G. Klein, 1970.
3 Ross, 1999, p. 99.
4 Ross, 1999, p. 93.
5 Ross, 1999, p. 94.
6 Rosen, 1974, pp. 189–209.
7 Ross, 1999, p. 96.
8 Ross, 1999, p. 97.
9 Ross, 1999, p. 97.
10 Ross, 1999, p. 97.
11 See Part I, Chapter 6, "Thomas Ogden and privacy on the couch".
12 See Part I, Chapter 7, "Christopher Bollas and the evocative couch".
13 See Part I, Chapter 12, "James Grotstein's dramaturgical and neuropsychic couch".

Chapter 14

Other authors and different approaches to psychoanalytic work from the couch

This penultimate chapter of Part I is intended to bring new bibliographical references not previously mentioned, and also to share reflections by authors who, in most cases, lack publications in Portuguese. Certainly, there are Brazilian psychoanalysts discussing the functions of the couch and the dichotomy of couch *versus* face-to-face, but because the Brazilian reader can find them more easily (at least when compared to foreign bibliographical references), the choice was not to include them here, leaving it up to the reader to carry out this research.

It's impossible to have everything. Therefore, it is also a fact that many foreign contributions end up being left out, since I have favoured positions taken from the original texts of the authors with whom I was able to have direct contact, rather than comments from others. The following notes include contributions by authors who are better known to the Brazilian public, as well as those who are not so well known. Throughout the chapter, the reader will find contributions from Otto Rank, Karl Abraham, Otto Fenichel, Michael Balint, Donald Meltzer, Masud Khan, Jean Laplanche, César and Sara Botella, Paula Heimann, Hanna Segal, Antonino Ferro, among others. Some of the contributions are very specific, but they reinforce the need to problematise the functions of the couch and its theoretical and clinical implications. For my part, I would like to point out in advance that the contributions by Danielle Quinodoz and Richard Waugaman seem particularly interesting in relation to the discussion proposed in the previous chapters. However, all the positions presented here will help to problematise what has been presented above.

The intention of this chapter is not to discuss each author's contribution in depth, as was done in most of the previous chapters, but to offer them to the reader as possibilities for understanding the couch. As such, this chapter serves more as a collage of vignettes, gathering different perspectives on the couch, so that the reader can assimilate and criticise them on the basis of their experience and their reading of the previous chapters. From this perspective, this chapter is not divided into sub-chapters. It will be one large text, separated by intervals, with the name of the author who contributed to our theme highlighted in bold, marked in this way as anchors to facilitate the reader's research.

DOI: 10.4324/9781003681212-16

* * *

The vast majority of the contributions here originally come from the English language. However, let's start with the French-language contributions. In *The Tina: The Transcendence of Transference*,[1] **Jean Laplanche** emphasises the importance of Freud's observation that the use of the couch was a "vestige of the hypnotic method", since the hypnotic method was, in itself, an inducer of transference and infantile regression, as well as a suppression of the outside world (in the hypnotic method, Freud asked the patient to close their eyes) and as a promoter of relaxation intended to "privilege the fantasy world".[2] The use of the couch in analysis would then be, for Laplanche, a severe trial against voyeurism – which would play a major role in neuroses – and a way of isolating transference from concrete intrusion.

Laplanche points out that there are three aspects that justify the use of the couch: (1) for him, there is a symbolic distinction between lying down and standing up, there is a "postural materialisation" of what comes from its psychic functioning; (2) the couch excludes a certain type of communication that involves the act of seeing, suggesting that psychoanalytic communication necessarily involves speech; (3) there is a positional dissymmetry between analyst and analysand, "one being in the visual field of the other and the other not being seen".[3] "It is in this way that the *distinction between the lying position and the standing* or 'face to face' *position* can, in effect, be considered as a true symbolic materialisation of the analytic situation, with its temporal-spatial wall."[4]

However, Laplanche goes on to tell us about non-verbal communication, also based on the use of the couch, and reinforces that, when lying down, only the analysand is deprived of looking at the other. He goes back to Freud and his clinical cases to say that the analyst is not deprived of seeing the analysand and their bodily movements (unconscious communications manifested by their body), which would be non-verbal communications. He therefore reiterates that the experience of analysing on the couch takes non-verbal signs into account. "On the couch, the patient speaks, but they don't just speak, they don't just say words," says **Christophe Dejours**,[5] a psychoanalyst who works in the field of psychosomatics and who also comments:

> The theory of the seduction of the child by the adult, revised and expanded by Laplanche, is also a way of revisiting and deepening the concept of the couch-armchair analytical device and the transference, with this exegesis that leads to the notion of "hollow transference". A transference designed to receive the enigma as the *sine qua non of* perlaboration, in other words, of the translation–de-translation–re-translation movement. Transference that recognises that the essence of interpretation originates in the patient himself, while the analyst strives to work above all with frustration (*Versagung*).[6]

Jacques André,[7] in returning to the discussion about the use of the couch or face-to-face, tells us about a clinical case in which the analysand had suffered physical aggression on his face (more precisely in his mouth, causing him to lose his teeth):

> With this patient I had asked myself the question: on the couch or face to face? Each answer had its drawbacks. The lying position, more than the loss of vision it brings, would be fearful because of the possibility of a schizoid return, as well as the threat of persecution. Lorenzo's homosexuality added a zone of uncertainty, between the eroticisation of "behind" and the argument of paranoid risk. But face to face contained a destructive visual violence, which he made immediately recognisable. He had re-done his teeth and imagined that his interlocutor was only looking at his teeth, which were as white as they were false. Later, he would evoke group scenes: just as he was talking "spontaneously", he suddenly caught an oblique gaze that coldly "laid him bare", an "entomological" gaze that penetrated him savagely and "rooted him out".

André evokes the risk of a paranoid emergence from the use of the couch, but in the end he indicates it, under the prerogative that it would be better for the analysand to "imagine" taking punches (the ones he had already taken traumatically), rather than "receiving them in the face", which would happen psychically from face-to-face.

In a 1999 interview[8] about the couch, **Jacques-Alain Miller** makes poetic comments about its function:

> Oh yes, the couch is a kind of bed. It's a bed that has no interior: you don't slip on the sheets, you lie on a surface. Like a reclining figure, with the deadly evocations that can surround it. As in the Baudelaire verse: "couches as deep as tombs". The bed is usually the place where one finds one's own body, the body that has been forgotten in active life, and where one also finds the body of the other. The couch, on the other hand, is a single bed. It makes the sexual relationship present and, at the same time, manifests its absence. Perhaps we could say that the couch is a changing room where the body is put on, where the active body is stripped off, where the imaginary body, the self-image, is also left behind. What remains is a third body, the body that is our rags, that rubbish that the subject drags behind him and that is so dear to him.
>
> As furniture, the couch is as important as Samuel Beckett's rubbish bin. It embodies the following paradox: you have to bring your body to the session and, at the same time, you have to undress it. The couch is a machine, a multiguillotine, which amputates the body of its motricity, its ability to act, its upright posture, its visibility. It materialises the abandoned body, the harvested body, the slaughtered body. To lie on the couch is to become a

> pure speaker, experiencing oneself as a body parasitised by speech, a poor body sick with the disease of speakers.

He concludes by criticising online consultations as non-psychoanalytical, also commenting – without further explanation – that the use of the couch is indicated in some cases and not in others.

* * *

Among the earliest contributions to the subject, we find that of **Melitta Schmideberg**, Melanie Klein's eldest daughter and one of the pioneers in thinking about early childhood deprivation and the psychoanalytic treatment of criminals. Schmideberg was a severe critic of her mother, above all because Klein's theory and technique focused exclusively on the internal world, without taking into account environmental factors in psychic development. She sided with Anna Freud against Klein in the British controversies. For Schmideberg, a "firm but sensitive" analytic style would help the analysand feel more secure in expressing their anxieties. In her clinical work, we see reports of analysands urinating on the couch, as well as analysands refusing to lie down.[9] Writing about claustrophobia,[10] Schmideberg even comments that the anxieties mobilised on the couch could obstruct the psychoanalytic process, which is also a veiled criticism of her mother's technique. Considerations about the couch as a negative mobiliser of phobic analysands are followed up by **Otto Fenichel**:

> As a rule, we don't give in to resistance, but we do analyse it. However, there are some exceptions: if a patient has agoraphobia, we won't demand that they forget their fear and go out into the street before the analysis begins. We have to calculate the extent to which the patient can resist the restrictions of their phobia. If we get the impression that a patient can't lie down and would rather be without the analysis, we should allow them to sit down. Then we must be very careful not to allow them to feel the phobic avoidance as a new (false) sense of security; we should insist that people talk about it. Secondly, the patient may feel anxious when lying down. The magical character of lying down can be used for resistance in such a way that analysis and life become isolated from each other and the patient vaguely feels that what they say when they are lying down has no validity when they are standing up. Some patients who are shy in other situations are uninhibited on the couch. So it may seem that an analysis is going well, but this is only true when the patient is lying down. Using this position exclusively can nullify the effectiveness it usually has. Just as some patients go to the toilet before or after analysis time, or perform some special act that separates analysis time from the rest of their lives, for others the external situation of analysis serves the same purpose. The analyst must interpret the resistance to this. In many cases, we support the interpretation by making the patient feel and realise how differently they experience the new situation.

> Communicating that the analysis can also be carried out with the patient sitting down is often enough for the patient to realise that for them "analysis" and "reality" are different and that a change in posture is not necessary. Freud pointed out how important it is to thwart the intention of some patients to divide the analytical interview into two parts, one "official" and the other "unofficial", when the patient says a few more words to the analyst after the hour is up. This attempt, according to Freud, should be thwarted by the analyst's introduction of the "unofficial" sentences in the next "official" session. But just as often, the opposite measure must be applied to eliminate resistance through isolation. Continuing, even for a moment, with a conversation or an interpretation that began at the moment of analysis, when the patient is no longer lying down, is very effective proof that analysis includes the whole of the individual's life, even when the patient is not lying on the couch.[11]

In his 1941 book *Problems of Psychoanalytic Technique*,[12] Fenichel works in a border zone between Freud's thoughts and those of Ferenczi. He remains attached to the former's technical indications, which include a certain "principle of frustration" of internal impulses, but he also takes into account the latter's clinical contributions, such as the notions of relaxation and elasticity. In his conception, the couch allows for a certain "relaxation" of the analysand, due to the impossibility seeing the analyst, thus avoiding entering a state of surveillance of his facial expressions. However, as in the quote used, he opens himself up to thinking about possibilities for abandoning the couch, if that seems worthwhile.

For **Balint**,[13] the analysand's relationship with the couch can have certain stages. In some, there may be feelings of attachment, of security; in others, there may be great mistrust. For him, there is an intermediate phase in which there is a moment when the analysand wants to leave the couch (which he allows, when necessary), out of fear and/or curiosity (about the analyst), trying to test his patience and tolerance. In this phase, the analyst is perceived as a dangerous object and the object world as hostile. It would only be after oscillations that the analysand would really trust the work from the couch, relaxing their posture, "turning on their side, curling up or asking for a blanket".

For Balint, it would only be at the last stage of treatment that the analysand would be able to "close his eyes and wrap himself in its protection, cosiness, darkness without structure" (referring to the couch). Only then would the analysand be able to enter and leave, at the beginning and end of the session, and move between the world of the couch and the world in which they put "the weight back on [their] … own shoulders – without great joy, but without bitter resentment". Balint states that: "the baby begins its existence – like our patients – mainly lying on their backs … When we start treatment, we offer our patients a configuration that in almost all cases induces them to adopt an infantile posture."[14] Without failing to mention the entry into regressive states, subjective experiences felt like "shipwrecks", in which the analysand feels like they are sinking, Balint also tells us about experiences of feeling "submerged" and, above all, experiences of feeling in states of fusion.

Karl Abraham[15] describes analysands closing their eyes on the couch and "describing mental images that came to mind",[16] relating them to dreams. These images would contain latent meanings, infantile, unconscious contents to be explored. Abraham reports analysands who take inanimate objects from the analyst's room as representatives of these fantasies, citing examples that would involve contents related to sexuality, both pre-oedipal and genital.[17] He tells us of the vision of analysands becoming blurred as bodily excitations emerged, which would be hysterical attacks dramatised in session to be worked through – symptomatic linked to the neurotic conflict of infantile sexuality.

Otto Rank,[18] in turn, associates the analytical situation and the use of the couch as representative of an intrauterine state, taking analytical work as a reliving of the time spent in the womb, with analysis being a kind of rebirth, emphasising the transferential relationship of a maternal nature, rather than the paternal relationship, or the Oedipal conflict itself –preponderant in Freudian thought until then.

* * *

In a 1948 text, **Adolph Stern**[19] raised questions about the use of the couch versus face-to-face work with borderline analysands, supporting his practice on the real materiality of the session to the detriment of the transference arising from past experiences. He comments that, when treated on the couch, his borderline analysands were usually withdrawn and distant, remaining "guarded against the involvement of affective transference, as well as against other affective manifestations. There were voluminous associations, apparently 'free' but obviously biased, based on the need to win over the analyst".[20] Stern implies in his text that he used to be more passive in these treatments, just like in an analysis of neurotics, because, based on his observations about the use of the couch in these cases, he affirmed the need for the analyst to be more active, moving these consultations to face-to-face. According to him, "The analyst couldn't stay out of the lives and feelings of these patients", in order to work through their capacity for object love. Stern points out that the sitting position "is the usual position in ordinary friendly relationships" and that this position would help the analyst to better observe the behaviour and facial expressions of the analysand, while they would be "less inclined to believe that the analyst is a possessor of mysteries, inaccessible, and the bearer of taboos".

Beyond this, Stern even mentions allowing an analysand to touch his arm, trying to show that he wasn't an inaccessible analyst or that he represented an authoritarian figure, under the pretext of working the session more from reality than from the reactions of a "previous and unreal transference". Stern relies on the idea that these analysands fear the rejections they experienced in childhood and that a new atmosphere must be created between analyst and analysand, so that the latter feels that the analyst is not disrespectful, but genuinely interested, and that he is supportive and protective of them.

The analyst would work to meet the needs of the analysand, since the real materiality of the session is what would work for the health of analysand, in other words, a "supportive therapy", according to his own words, in which "In the course of treatment, his/her capacity for objectal love relationships in his/her environment increases significantly".[21]

Victor Eisenstein, in a 1951 paper,[22] follows Adolph Stern's line of thought regarding borderline analysands, defending three fundamental points for these treatments: (1) the need for strong, human support from the analyst; (2) avoiding the free association technique of classical analysis; (3) preferably using the sitting position. He states: "In these disorders, the therapist must therefore assume the active and benevolent role of a parent, rather than the usual neutral position of an impersonal analyst; however, he must provide more than supportive or educational help."[23] In Eisenstein's view, referring this patient to the couch would accentuate his masochistic and dependent attitudes and exaggerate the "fantasised (projected) omnipotence" in the analyst, This would lead to a feeling that the analyst would not be "perceived as representing the reality that he or she should be",[24] and it is important to avoid regressive situations, stating that one cannot treat borderline states as one would treat a transference neurosis.[25]

Still on the subject of borderline disorders, **Gerald Adler**[26] published a work in 1988 that spoke of gradations of the disorder, even questioning its concept, arguing that such form of suffering present themselves in mixed configurations in relation to other psychopathological structures. Therefore, their understanding of the indication of the couch varies according to the seriousness of each case presented.

There are many studies[27] that discuss, based on various bibliographical references, issues concerning borderline disorders and, consequently, the indication (or not) of the couch in such cases. With the exception of one or two singular points, we could say that these positions tend to be more homogeneous.

* * *

Antonino Ferro, despite trying to understand the psychoanalytic process and the psychoanalytic technique as analogous to the dream, works most of his clinical cases face-to-face. He points out the excessive asymmetry resulting from the use of the couch and ironically states that what would make analytical work impossible is the analyst's superego.[28] Ferro also describes an appointment in which an analysand was in the armchair while the analyst was lying on the couch, arguing that **Marie Bonaparte**, when she suffered from rheumatism, conducted her sessions in this way.[29]

As for the role of the couch in psychoanalytic work, **Leo Sadow**[30] and **Anton Kris**[31] each point out, in their own way, how working on the couch facilitates a certain relaxation and sharpening of the senses for listening to the analysand's material. Leo Sadow explains how the face-to-face modality, despite bringing more sensory elements to the analyst's work, it saturates their senses, making it difficult to sharpen their listening skills. Kris, for his part, points out that, at first, the couch can mobilise anxieties in the analysand, sometimes awakening transferences of a parental nature in which the analysand might feel subjected to a hierarchical order, but, as they experience the work on the couch, this could dissipate, leading the analysand to relaxation, which aids the process of free association.

Ernst Wolf,[32] in addition to what we have discussed elsewhere, points out that Freud's use of the couch was intended to isolate the transference, to allow it to emerge in due course, defined as resistance. Wolf comments that the use of the couch would be a way of facilitating the emergence of archaic or infantile ways of psychic organisation, often related to infantile sexuality, relative dependence and helplessness, which would be actualised transferentially in order to facilitate analytical treatment. The similarity to the position of the bed can lead to associations related to "bedtime" fantasies, and archaic traumas can be recalled that would not be accessible without the regressive propensities of using the couch.

In the case of a fragile *self*, the analysand may regress with such intensity and demand too much of the analyst that, even using all their efforts, they may tire of exercising the caring functions demanded by the analysand's *self*, causing the work to stagnate, or leading hateful and destructive tendencies on the part of the analysand to erupt. Since it is part of the analyst's job to support and adequately handle the demands of the analysand's fragile self, Wolf advises against inexperienced analysts conducting more regressive analyses on the couch. Despite this, Wolf also points out how working face-to-face would tire the analyst and their listening efforts, which stem from the effort to contain their natural bodily reactions to the analysand's communications. He points out that even on the couch and not having access to the analyst's expressions, the analysand would be picking up his presence and what would be the analyst's persona, his tone of voice, his bodily noises. His perspective is that the choice of each intervention and word uttered by the analyst influences the analytical work, indicating that isolating the transference, in order to maintain neutrality, is something that belongs to the realm of the impossible – and that Freud certainly knew this very well. The transference, then, would also be moulded by what is expressed by the analyst, regardless of what form it takes.

In more serious cases, Wolf comments that the regression facilitated by the use of the couch can precipitate disintegrative processes that affect the cohesion of the *self*. Therefore, each case must be assessed individually, and some borderline cases could benefit from the couch. However, he points out that some neurotics may resist the couch and insist on being treated face-to-face because of some inhibition or phobia, or even because they feel humiliated by the referral. It would be necessary to think about the feelings of submission related to parental figures, which would be directed to the analyst when referring them to the couch.

* * *

Danielle Quinodoz[33] is original in her thinking, preferring not to use the nomenclature borderline to the detriment of what she would call heterogeneous analysands – analysands who have not managed to integrate their *self*. Her theoretical-clinical proposal involves conceiving the psychic experience without detaching oneself from the order of the body and the sensory. Her listening and intervention aim at fostering the integration of the self, while at the same time involving the body in this process. Thus, the sensory perception and the sensory countertransference, which are felt in the analyst's body, become auxiliaries to listening and to intervention. Thus, she carries her expression "words that touch" to its ultimate consequences.

Quinodoz understands that the couch amplifies the analysand's awareness of their bodily experiences. Eliminating the visual experience with the analyst would lead the analysand to focus on their internal/corporeal experiences to the detriment of external stimuli. Visual access to the psychoanalyst can impede the development of the transference. The inability to see the analyst's facial expressions and bodily movements makes it easier for the analysand to better explore the analyst's interventions.

Quinodoz states that there are analysands who are capable symbolising and using neurotic mechanisms, and who, without actually being psychotic, make use of primitive mechanisms characteristic of psychosis, such as denial, projection and massive projective identification, among other varied forms of splitting/divisions. The internal heterogeneity of these analysands, which we could understand as the result of splits, does not allow them to integrate themselves as a whole. Therefore, Quinodoz's interventions, her words to the analysand, are designed and intended to talk to both the more neurotic and the more psychotic side of the analysand, criticising analysts who only address one of the "sides" of the analysand. In her view, the analyst will only find the words to "touch" the analysand if they allow themselves to be "touched" in their guts by the language of the analysand. Therefore, her intervention is based on "a form of language that is not restricted to the verbal transmission of thoughts, but incorporates feelings and the sensations that accompany these feelings".[34] The repercussions of the analyst's interventions, when they manage to achieve the aim of enunciating "words that touch", give the feeling that there is a human interlocution in its entirety. "[L]anguage that touches", Quinodoz states,

> is an *embodied* language. Patients who are distressed by their lack of internal cohesion need to be heard by an analyst who listens to them with the whole body of their *self* included – and who addresses the totality of their person when talking to them – again, including the body. The analyst's language can serve as a vehicle for the analysand. That's why, for example, in cases

> where I choose to tell a patient the fundamental rule at the beginning of an analysis, instead of using the traditional formula, "say everything that comes to mind", I simply say, "say everything that comes …" I don't want to prioritise the mind, and I leave the patient free to continue the sentence internally as they see fit. It's up to them to feel not only what comes, but also where it comes from.[35]

For Quinodoz,[36] the analytic *setting* allows for non-verbal communication and allows the split-off parts of the analysand to take their place on the couch. She states that the criterion of analysability is usually thought of by most analysts only from the point of view of the analysand – whether they would be able to enter an analysis process – but that this criterion should also be thought of from the point of view of the analyst. The author argues that analysability depends on the analyst's ability to listen and intervene, and she declares herself deeply indignant when she hears analysts reporting drowsiness or sudden episodes of falling asleep while listening to their analysands during sessions, since this constitutes a disservice to psychoanalysis.

Felix Deutsch, Helene Deutsch's husband, in his 1952 text "Analytical Posturology",[37] focused on thinking in detail about the movements and body positions of his analysands, including their relationship with the couch, based on various clinical reports. His work emphasises bodily communications and their meanings, which often precede verbal communications, reinforcing verbal communications (or contradicting them), manifesting unconscious contents beyond what words can achieve. When lying on the couch, the movements and positions of the legs, hands and arms would be the analysand's unconscious communications of all kinds, and could manifest issues linked to orality, anality, situations linked to trauma, primary motility, the expression of oedipal contents and various conflicts. The analysand's free associations are also corporeal and can be "listened to".

In metapsychological terms, Felix Deutsch states that a psychic stimulus presses for a discharge and "a functional organic process", initiated by the stimulus, which leads to a "postural rearrangement that continues and completes the psychological process". Consequently, he states "that the amount of physiological discharge corresponds to the amount of emotion not discharged, until it is exhausted".[38] **James McLaughlin**[39] corroborates Felix Deutsch and, also through clinical details, reflects on bodily movements and positions on the couch, which are impossible to exemplify here without dwelling on the singularity of the cases he presents.

* * *

Donald Meltzer[40] contributes to the theme of the couch, often metaphorically associating it with the uterus, but also with the penis, breasts and other elements of Kleinian theory. Beyond the couch, Meltzer is concerned with thinking about the analysand's relationship with the consulting room as a whole. He stresses his habit of closing his eyes while listening to the analysand, sporadically monitoring their bodily movements and facial expressions from a diagonal orientation of the couch. He states:

> The person on the couch is an absolute stranger who is not displaying their personality, but only their techniques for adapting to the claustrophobic world they inhabit. At the moment when an analyst can recognise the quality of imprisonment and the essential struggle for survival in an uninhabitable situation, he sees a child who has lost himself, moved away from home, who has even forgotten the qualities of the home he once knew, perhaps in the most serious cases only the womb.[41]

Throughout his work, Meltzer also shows us the couch playing transferential roles in the analysis of children, as well as reporting cases of adolescents in which the couch is used in the mould of adults. Regarding the analysis of adolescents, he describes periods of transition in which, on entering puberty, these analysands would use the couch and the analysis room in a mixed way – sometimes this happens in conjunction with children's play; at other times, these analysands lie on the couch and make associations, just like adults. Among his clinical examples, we find regressive uses of the couch that involve experiences with the mother's body and breast, sometimes with the analysand covering themselves on the couch, etc.[42] On the treatment of adults, he writes the following passage, alluding to the function of bodily gestures that are allied to the expression psychic materials:

> Although it is not part of my technique to comment on a patient's behaviour on the couch or to ask them for associations, scrutinising posture and movement patterns and linking them to dream material sometimes allows for a fruitful interpretation of behaviour. In this way, the series of modifications of anal masturbation can be revealed and a more successful search for real anal stimulation instituted. For example, a patient who often kept both hands in his pockets recognised through a dream that this was sometimes accompanied by pulling at a loose thread. This led to the perception that he had the habit of manually plucking the perianal hairs before defecation so that they would not spoil the shape of his emerging faecal matter."[43]

Alessandro Bruni[44] comments that the sensory deprivation present in the use of the couch and the fact that the analysand explores the analyst's actual physical presence can produce, in the psychotic part of the personality, an "unbearable decrease in 'material for thinking', material that is mainly made up of those non-verbal products of the analyst that accompany the interpretative activity, such as expressions of the eyes, changes in facial expression, muscle tensions and movements, changes in tone of voice, etc.".[45] However, despite this, Bruni relates a clinical case in which he exemplifies the importance of the couch for accessing this psychotic part of oneself.

Bruni tells us about a clinical case in which he suspected that his analysand – on the couch – was entering a hallucinatory stupor and that, when he said something to the analysand – Bruni doesn't remember exactly what the analysand said – in order to reassure him of his presence, Bruni got the following response: "Doctor, thank you for talking to me! It was terrible! The space around me was expanding and the distance between the objects in that space kept growing. In the end, you were so far away in infinite space that I was about to lose you"[46] – a situation experienced in analysis that was a milestone in the disappearance of the analysand's agoraphobia. In Bruni's view, a kind of epiphany occurred, based on entering a great vacuum, which took the analysand out of object existence, but which was fundamental for a process of benign and reparative reintrojection. Still on this case, Bruni reports that the analysand occasionally experienced motor agitations and terror on the couch, with moments of confusion, which diminished as the analysis progressed. According to Bruni, this occurred because the analysand, during the process of analysis, was removing "false prostheses" from his real *self*.

Angelika Staehle[47] describes an analysand who frequently struggled with claustrophobic, persecutory and psychosomatic issues and strong anxieties on the couch, spending a long time describing his body states, his sensations and his hypochondriacal anxieties in order to work on them. This same analysand even got a job near the analyst's office and during his working hours, would park his car in front of the office window. Staehle saw this as way for the analysand to concretely signal that he didn't want her to "let him out of her sight". The analyst understood the case as a dependent *self*. She understood that the analysand manifested, in some way, in his dreams and in his sessions, "the cry of a baby for help". The couch (and the analyst's room as a whole, perhaps even the car park in front of the consulting room window), in this case, also served as a depository containing the anxieties arising from the analysand's psyche.

In addition to the case mentioned above, Staehle also tells us about a child[48] who, in his own way, used the couch as an object to help him work. At the beginning of his analysis, this 5-year-old boy would hide under the couch, saying he didn't want to be found, and would remain there incommunicado, which led the analyst to understand the boy's act as related to a couch-mother transference, like that of a baby who wanted to return to its mother's womb to be born again. At this point in the treatment, the analyst would be seen as an object that was separate from him and with which he couldn't yet relate.

Still on the subject of analysing children, **Joshua Durban**[49] recounts scenes of an analysand on the autistic spectrum who manifested herself by lying curled in the foetal position on the couch, with blankets covering her head, as one of the other ways of manifesting herself in session. **Angela Sowa**, **Geneviève Haag**, **Anne Alvarez** and **Bianca Lechevalier-Haïm**,[50] who basically deal with autistic suffering, also report on the use that children can make of the couch during their analyses. **Frances Tustin**,[51] who worked with children on the autistic and/or psychotic spectrum, has written about cases in which they, the child analysands, use the couch to fulfil masturbatory fantasies, as well as to work on issues involving contact with themselves.

Sydney Klein, **Didier Houzel** and **Judith Mitrani**[52] think about the emergence of autistic states in the analysis of adults, and how these manifestations present themselves on the couch. Many of their examples are less explicit and difficult to present in a few words, but one of Judith Mitrani's cases is more didactic.

As well as Mitrani reporting analysands falling asleep, among other situations, she tells us of a case in which an analysand covered herself with the blanket at the foot of the couch during every session, even on hot days. Mitrani noticed that, by doing this, the analysand was trying to connect with her body in a private way, trying to hide as much as possible from the analyst but, over time, she could notice that the analysand sometimes sucked her own thumb, as well as caressing her body in a masturbatory way. Part of the analytic work involved tolerating such behaviours until it was possible to work on them verbally.

According to Mitrani,[53]

> an environment of relative safety and security needs to be maintained. Our consulting rooms are likened, in the unconscious, to the mother's body. Furthermore, just as the modulation of the ups and downs of the mother's emotional and mental state and her physicality are essential for healthy foetal development and the baby's exit from the womb, for adult patients the therapeutic setting and the rhythm and consistency of the work affect development, the ability to unite and separate healthily.

* * *

Hanna Segal presents us with clinical cases of schizophrenia that use the couch in different ways. In one of the cases,[54] she tells us about a treatment in which an analysand used the couch in a similar way to that used in the analyses of children. This person used the room as a whole, with the couch being used sporadically by her to lie down – and even masturbate – as well as to try to express a kind of unconscious reliving linked to her suffering. Another clinical case of schizophrenia was treated along the lines of a classic treatment, which was very successful, since the analysand developed very well, with important gains for his life. In this second case,[55] Segal avoided confronting the analysand's delusions and hallucinations. She comments:

> In the sixth month of treatment, the formal analytical situation was finally established. The patient was lying on the couch, associating and, at least

> consciously, didn't expect anything from me apart from analysis. From then on, my problems were the same as those of the analysis of a neurotic, that is, the analysis of the patient's system of fantasies and defences.[56]

According to Segal, the analysand continued to live with pathology, but developed his life to the point where he had important professional achievements and managed to start a family.

Francis Baudry[57] tells us of an analysand who, lying on the couch, shouted violently at him. His aggression really frightened the analyst, and even colleagues from other rooms in the building called him to say that the shouting was interfering with their work. One day, during his analysis, this analysand positioned himself on the couch, lying on his side with one foot out on the floor, and gave an immense, terrifying scream (a "blood-curdling" scream, says Baudry). The analysand then said: "This is what I heard as a baby, when my defective sister screamed at the top of her lungs, terrifying me."[58] This manifestation became a way of signifying the terror that the analysand was making the analyst feel and, consequently, began to provide elements for analysing the trauma.

Judy Eekhoff[59] tells us the story of an analysand whose suffering was not linked to her emotions, and there was a disconnection between the mind and the body – something that Eekhoff realised. The analysand's posture on the couch and her long silences made the analyst imagine her lying in a coffin. Eekhoff commented: "Just as a mother is often 'combined' with the breathing of her breastfed baby, I found myself breathing with her,"[60] often imagining her as a baby. As the analysis progressed, Eekhoff witnessed more spontaneous bodily gestures, as well as many criticisms and attacks directed at her as analyst, in addition to the presentation of confusional states, perhaps even delusions and hallucinations, consisting of the idea that the analyst might strangle her.

The analysand alternated between paranoid moments and moments of fusion, leading the analyst to extreme countertransference states, to the point where she considered totally doubting her technical abilities and even psychoanalysis. However, according to Eekhoff's detailed reports, the analysis was increasingly showing signs of being on the right track, and what was experienced in session began to be worked out in favour of the analysand's psychic health.[61]

Ofra Eshel[62] commented that if the analyst doesn't dedicate themself to connecting with the analysand's suffering and reaching them in their primitive states, the couch will become an insurmountable "iron cradle".

Celia Korbivcher,[63] when looking at non-integrated states of the psyche (the work of analysis being to integrate them), brings us a clinical vignette that alludes to the transference that can be directed towards the couch. The author mentions an analysand who lay on her stomach, seeking bodily comfort, staring at the wall and saying, among other things: "This is the only place I experience this. I come here and I cling tightly to this sofa ... I feel like I'm missing very basic things in my life ..." and, in a calm tone, "I look at the wall and think: 'Oh, my wall!' You know, I always look at the little dots on the wall and think that if I could, I'd rip them off the wall and take them with me, but I know I can't do that."[64]

* * *

Harold Kelmon,[65] **Jacob Jacobson,**[66] **John Gedo**[67] and **Marianne Goldberger**[68] discuss the advantages and disadvantages of using the couch, without it being possible to highlight anything that hasn't already been explained in this book at some point, except for the fact that Gedo advocates that there are pre-verbal communication gestures that can only be manifested face-to-face, while Kelmon focuses on the spatiality of the room, bodily movements and the countless positional arrangements of the analysand's body (on or off the couch), as often communicating more than the words that come from free association. **Neil Skolnick,**[69] writing from a "relational" perspective, focuses on the disadvantages of the couch and the therapeutic need for the gaze, arguing that the couch serves the analyst more than the patient and the therapeutic process, drawing on the positions of **Sullivan**, **Fromm**, **Lichtenberg**, **Fairbairn** and many other analysts.

Fairbairn[70] claims that the use of the couch is a remnant of the hypnotic technique, and that Freud used it because he didn't like being observed. His position is that analysts have found rationalisations to justify it and that, because of this, he, Fairbairn, wouldn't use it, advocating an intermediate spatial position in which the analysand, seated, could choose to look or not. Fairbairn[71] advocates this:

> the use of the couch imposes a taboo on any form of activity, except verbal expression; and since inhibitions about activities are such an important factor in the genesis of symptoms and inner difficulties, it is questionable whether the artificial reinforcement of such inhibitions by the conditions of the analytic session does not, in many cases, constitute a serious emotional trauma for the patient, increasing their resistance and perhaps even favouring negative therapeutic reactions. There are, of course, patients of the passive type for whom the reclining position on the couch provides a convenient escape from the anxiety involved in the activity, and who are all too ready to exploit the analytic situation in a masochistic way; and the question that arises in such cases is to what extent it is desirable for the conditions of analysis to provide the patient with such a ready means of escape, combined with such a convenient means of hidden masochistic gratification.[72]

In addition, there are other studies[73] that attempt to discuss the advantages and disadvantages of using the couch, using various bibliographical references, including many that we are working with here.

* * *

In her work on the nature and function of fantasy, **Susan Isaacs**[74] tells us about the function of the couch as a facilitator of the analyst's work, which allows her to capture "every detail of gesture or tone of voice, rhythm of speech and its variations", as well as "particular changes in the way of expressing oneself, changes in mood, every sign of affection or denial of affection", to manifest its nature and its particular intensities from the associative context. All these details would help her to unveil "unconscious fantasies (among other mental truths)", making them increasingly clear.

Harold F. Searles[75] recounts a scene of an analysand who, pathologically, was seen by him as falling within the spectrum of mixed neuroses. In a clinical vignette, he describes when the analysand said goodbye to the couch and not to the analyst. He said "Goodbye couch" and then, addressing the analyst, said: "Take good care of the couch after I leave." The analyst's understanding was that the couch was "carrying" the transference to the analyst and serving to express what the analysand, unable to say more directly – perhaps covering up a more direct transference –, wanted to communicate: "Goodbye, Searles, take care."

Searles also emphasises the use of the couch as a transitional object:

> As Searles (1976) pointed out, one transferential meaning that the couch can take on is that of a transitional object. He cites a patient who reacted intensely to his absences and who once said of his couch: "It's more real to me than you … I can't touch you, I can't do things with you. This couch here nice and safe." Searles goes on to comment: "As for the significance of the couch for me, if I think about my relationships with my various patients, I find it easy to believe that it often functions as a transitional object" (p. 557). Searles' hypothesis is pertinent to a patient who asked herself in a session: "Will part of the couch stick to me when I get up?" She then vigorously pulled on a tuft of fabric covering the sofa and remarked: "No, it won't come off …" On another occasion, this patient speculated that I put paper towels on the couch pillow "so that I could throw the patient away after the session".[76]

Greenson, in turn, relates the transference to inanimate objects, including the objects in the analyst's room, to transitional objects, being "The couch, its covers or anything else in the immediate area is often treated as a transitional object".[77]

* * *

The highly interesting text "*The Analytic Couch as a Transference Object*" (1995),[78] written by **Richard Waugaman**, points to the importance of pre-verbal communications, but goes beyond even this understanding. Through countless clinical vignettes, Waugaman demonstrates clinical situations in which the couch is taken as a transference object, amplifying the role that inanimate objects in the consulting room – especially the couch – can play in the transference field.

Waugaman follows Searles' perspective in which "The analytic couch is a central feature of the non-human environment within the analyst's room",[79] and brings up some clinical cases in which the analysands relate the couch to a bed and a bed's functions, linked to rest, sleep, dreaming and sexual intercourse.

I think it's interesting to bring up a clinical case by Waugaman, even though it lacks a few details. Waugaman presents us with a case in which the couch pillow occupies an unconscious fantasy of a mother's breast[80] for an analysand. The analysand never rested his head quietly on the pillow, always on his hands. According to Waugaman, his mother's post-natal depression and a breast abscess (which prevented the baby from suckling) led the analysand to an experience of distance, with the pillow as a transferential substitute. The fact that the analyst put a new paper towel on the couch pillow at the beginning of each session (for all the patients) helped to feed a transference in which the analysand felt afraid of damaging or dirtying the analyst's furniture. The analysand was just as worried about getting the couch dirty as he was about relating more spontaneously to his mother's breast. He was also afraid that the analyst would get distracted and not pay attention to his speech. His declared fear of dirtying the couch involved getting his shoes dirty, and he would even change his clothes before the sessions to make sure he didn't dirty the couch in any way. He was afraid of spoiling the analyst's object (the couch), or the analyst himself, often expressing a fear of "spreading his germs".

After two years of analysis and dealing with these issues, the analysand ends up resting his head on the pillow without the intermediary support of his hand. The first thing he reports when he does this is that his wife's breast was sore because it was full of milk, and, fearing that she might have an infection, he decides to suck her milk. The analysand says that without his hands on his head, he doesn't know what to do with them, just as he felt when he was a teenager. In addition, he was afraid that he would feel too comfortable leaving his head directly on the couch pillow – without putting his hands on it as an intermediary. For his part, Waugaman understands that the analysand had a fantasy of having done something bad to his mother.

> In his pre-Oedipal maternal transference, the pillow represented my breasts, which he was convinced would infect him with their dirty, hostile and sexual feelings. He defended himself against these fears with a variety of distancing manoeuvres. Resting his head on his hand was therefore a paradigmatic posture for him.[81]

The fact that the analyst put paper towels on couch pillow was experienced by the analysand as a non-acceptance of himself, involving feelings of being dirty and unwanted, as if the analyst wanted to get away from him. Having sucked his wife's milk, even when immersed in fantasies of infecting her, turned out to be an act of reparation in relation to his mother-baby fantasies.

The paper towel, placed on the couch by the analyst, evoked competition and rivalry in some other analysands, a reminder that other analysands always come and go. Waugaman mentions cases in which analysands toyed with the idea of leaving pins hidden under the couch pillow – intending to attack the next analysands who rested there, wanting to be the only ones to occupy the space.

Waugaman also reports on analysands who had some material related to death and guilt, either from relatives and loved ones or from themselves, and who ended up associating the couch with a coffin at some point. Others associated it with a surgical bed. **Harry Guntrip**[82] is another psychoanalyst who reported a clinical case in which an analysand, who had lost his father at an early age, had a "coffin" transference with the couch, identifying himself with his deceased father. There is also a clinical report involving fantasies of returning to the womb and links between the couch and the sexual act.[83]

Waugaman also brings up cases in which the couch is implicitly or explicitly experienced as a cradle, through reports, free associations or dreams. Among the examples is that of an analysand who felt physically "different" on the couch, "rocked as if in a cradle". Waugaman suggests that a "uterine transference" can emerge onto the analyst's couch: "Lying on the couch promotes a pre-Oedipal maternal transference, with unconscious fantasies of being in the arms or womb of the analyst."[84] To exemplify his comment, he brings up an analysand's dream about a kangaroo baby and its mother, which, in the work of analysis, was related by the analysand to the couch and its "pocket" at the bottom, formed by a certain envelope that protects the couch from the shoes of the analysands – also reinforcing his understanding of a possible transferential use of the couch as a womb, based on other examples.

In other cases, the work on the couch could refer to anality, and the couch as a kind of toilet. Among Waugaman's examples, there is a clinical vignette from **Gabbard** (1991)[85] in which the analysand says: "I have a fantasy of vomiting on your floor or defecating on your couch. I want to get rid of all that. I hate it when I can't provoke you into taking my anger. So I have to accept it. I need a place to dump. I've been using you as a pay toilet." One of Waugaman's analysands told him: "I felt we stopped before I was finished, like having to stop in the middle of a bowel movement – having to hold it back in until later." Another analysand, afraid of losing control over her sexual arousal, and who had recently experienced an episode of enuresis at a stressful time, says: "I just had a terrible thought – what if I wet the couch!?!? That would be the worst thing that could happen!", also alluding to the sexual nature of "getting wet".

One analysand, when she started lying on the couch, said that she was only used to lying on her back when she had sex, but not when she slept. Waugaman[86] comments: "**Rose** (1962)[87] and **Flournoy** (1979)[88] have suggested that patients may unconsciously see the beginning of treatment as a sexual act in which the analyst fertilises/impregnates them, as if it were repeating the primordial scene in which the patient was conceived." Among the cases reported was that of an analysand who really wanted to have a couch like his analyst's in his home and, because of this, did a lot of research. His justification was that "he was in love with the couch" and wanted to have it in his home environment too, adding that he would also like to use it for sexual encounters with women – perhaps denoting a kind of transference of desire and confirmation of potency through furniture.

According to Waugaman, there are analysands who see working on the couch as the place where their secrets will be revealed. He tells us of a case in which an analysand once lifted the carpet under one of the couch's feet to see if there was anything there, and then told the analyst that he wanted to know if there was anything "unpleasant" hidden there (as a kind of projection of what he himself was trying to hide from the analyst). The desire to possess the analyst's couch, in this case, "expressed his central fantasy of paternal transference, in which I would provide him with a superior phallus",[89] says Waugaman.

* * *

Masud Khan[90] was a controversial and important psychoanalyst who eventually succumbed to alcoholism and was overtaken, it seems, by paranoia and psychosis. There are many reports of analysands being extremely grateful to him as a great analyst and a determining factor in their lives. In Khan's conception, the couch would be available to be used in a relaxed way, while the *setting* as a whole would be a guardian of privacy, protecting the analysand from intrusions and violations of the outside world. In addition to neuroses, Khan dealt clinically and theoretically with the processes of integration of the *self* and regression processes under analysis, making the couch an important aid.[91]

One analysand compares Khan's consulting room to Winnicott's: "The room was dark, and I experienced it as cosy and like a womb, in contrast to Winnicott's open and clear space."[92] As for his clinical practice, we know that he allowed his analysands to choose (and change positions) between the couch and the armchair in front of the analyst.[93] Although Khan led his analysands to regress to dependency, especially in cases of false *self*, as his analyst Winnicott did, he claims never to have reached this stage in his long analysis. Khan reports that only three times during the period of his own analysis did he feel he was plunged deeply into himself, physically and psychosomatically. On one of these occasions, he says that he got off the couch and stuck his head down the side of Winnicott's jacket, and that the experience of listening to his heart led him to a great sense of peace, which remained vivid in his memory. As for the technique, he points out that Winnicott never interpreted this and the other occasions, allowing Khan to immerse himself to this point, so that his psyche could be "actualised".[94]

Another of Khan's analysands reports that at a certain moment, lying on the couch, she felt herself listening to her own voice, from her innermost being, and that it was from this experience that she found a feeling of great courage. Khan, impressed by the moment, moved towards her and embraced her.[95] In another account of an analysis conducted by Khan,[96] we find:

> As the analysis went on, I began to regress more and more. I curled up like a foetus under the blanket on Masud's sofa (he had a chequered blanket, which I think came from John Sutherland, who was Scottish). After a while, I regressed to something close to childhood. For at least a week, my experience of the ground was altered. It was as if I was a child learning to walk and wasn't sure my balance or where the ground was. It scared me – everything was just different and new. He gave me an extra session one weekend. I went into the room and immediately fell asleep on the couch. While I was asleep, I had a powerful dream that felt absolutely real. I dreamt that my whole body was enveloped by something of a different density to air – I was totally enveloped, like a maggot, by something that wasn't hard, but wasn't soft either. I felt totally at peace. In the dream state, there was a dog in the room, similar to a German shepherd my mum once had, and it was looking after me, watching over me. The dream continued without anything happening. I was there and the dog was near me. When I woke up, I came gently back to the present. I told Masud about the dream and he was completely quiet. We both knew that the dog in the dream was him. The word for "dog" in my native language is "can", which sounds the same as "Khan".
>
> This was a very important session, one that changed me. I used to get very depressed. I felt like I had a weight inside me and that it was making my life darker. After the session, I was never depressed like that again. The weight of that depression was gone and something was restored.

One of Khan's analysands[97] felt that, in some sessions, the analyst listened to him very well, while in others he didn't – perhaps already becoming aware of the analyst's mental decline. He also said that Khan was rude to him at times; that he took calls and drafted things that "certainly" had no connection to his analysis; and that his sessions were marked by interruptions from the analyst's secretary. Despite this, he recounted some good passages, including Khan's placing his hand on his head (on the couch) – which was very comforting, according to him – at a time when the analysand was very angry with his parents.

* * *

Bertram Lewin,[98] in 1955, commented that the couch could evoke fantasies of death, often associated with medical practice and operating tables, but also related to sleep. "Being put to sleep" as an act linked to health and healing – remembering that hypnosis (Freud's initial method) was seen as a "magical sleep", from which patients woke up cured/recovered. From this perspective, and reflecting on primary narcissism, the author relates "blank dreams" on the couch with "the baby", in its stage of primary narcissism, with primary care, the nurturing of the mother, the mother's body, and breastfeeding.

Comparing the work on the couch with the work of the dream, Lewin states that the formation of dreams can be equated with the formations that occur in the analytical situation,[99] citing a dream of Freud's, which Freud relates in *The Interpretation of Dreams*. In it, Freud was being dissected (like a corpse), in a dream-like presentation of his process of self-analysis – which we might associate with the couch and the curiosity to know oneself as deeply as possible. "The affections on the couch, or those that arise during solitary association, are like those that appear in dreams."[100] The analyst's role is to listen to "any human communication, from the most primitive to the most sophisticated".[101] He also recalls the importance of the musicality present in every communication.

Thus, Lewin relates the work on the couch to a "deep sleep", restorative and healing. For him, at certain stages of treatment, the musicality of the analyst's voice would be more important than the content of his words, in line with **Eissler**'s thinking.[102] For Lewin, the figure of the analyst, the transferential field, "surrounds" the work on the couch, in the same way that the outside world (the remains of the day, etc.) "surrounds" the dream.

Ida Macalpine[103] comments that the psychoanalytic *setting* and the use of the couch make the analysand present their childhood life. According to Macalpine, "the psychoanalytic technique creates an infantile *setting/scenario*" in which the analysand must adapt, albeit through regression. The analyst's neutrality and the indication of the couch "amount to a reduction of the analysand's object world and the denial of object relations in the room".[104] She ponders the fact that there is a deprivation of the object relation that restricts the conscious functions of the ego, encouraging a surrender to the pleasure principle and that, through their free associations, the analysand would end up being led to infantile reactions and attitudes, via transference. In other words, the analysand is not the only one responsible for their regression to the infantile, but the very indication of the couch and all the elements of the *setting* lead to this regression. For Macalpine, the analysing room is a safe place, even though it can evoke all kinds of anxieties at first. The restriction of the external object world; the lying down position; the constancy of an environment that stimulates fantasy and daydreaming; the indication that the analysand must give up any criticism of what arises in his thoughts; the fixed routine of a psychoanalytic "ceremonial", like a reminiscence of a disciplined childhood routine; the fact that the analysand does not receive a response from the analyst to his desires; and the frustration of gratifications – these would all be aimed at leading the analysand to a regression, into the realm of the infantile, creating an emotional state of ambivalence, in which their internal conflicts would present themselves – and this regression is what would make the analysands subsequently "grow up" in every sense.

For **Paula Heimann**, "only the baby is really a baby". Heimann argues[105] that regression is never complete, not even in the most severe psychoses, and that the child that presents itself through the adult in analysis is also not identical to the original child. For her, it is the horizontal position provided by the couch, added to the fundamental rule, as well as all the combinations of the situation that induce the emergence of the child. However, regression in analysis is never complete and is always mediated, in a way, by the adult side of the analysand, not least because the analyst is not in fact the father or mother of the analysand. Even if the analysand identified the analyst with their mother or breasts, the analysand would perceive the difference between their primary objects and the analyst, as well as perceiving personal characteristics of the analyst and the analytic encounter. Heimann[106] tells us of a case in which an analysand made use of the view out the window, through which the sky and the branches of the tree served as comfort, because she didn't live in a beautiful place. The analysand suggested that the analyst paint the room and its furniture white, like a nursery, taking the experience in analysis as a way of accessing a child's world, from a perspective mediated by adult experience, in order to develop a healthy narcissism that previously had no chance to emerge.

César and **Sara Botella**[107] argue that the regredience to a primary functioning of the psyche, provided by the couch, could lead to certain hallucinatory presentifications, even in non-neurotic analysands. An example of this would be smells that don't match material reality of the analysis session, but are consistent with the analysand's internal world.

Victor L. Schermer[108] emphasises that the use of the couch should not be seen as limiting or as a way of controlling variables, but rather has an evocative meaning, being an aid to maximum freedom of verbal expression, through free association, even opening up space for any type of manifestation – without these manifestations being repressed by the analyst. He points out that the analyst's "invisibility" does not make the process of analysis and the dynamics established something that only comes from the analysand, because the analyst is always sending verbal or non-verbal signals that affect the analysand, giving the example that the analysands end up producing dreams and fantasies that, in a way, "adapt to the analyst's theoretical orientation". Communication on preconscious levels is part of the psychoanalytic dynamic. Schermer also recalls the couch as an evocative of sexuality, as well as relating psychoanalytic dialogue as a kind of "dance" that takes place in the mother-baby interaction – based on Daniel Stern's contribution. For Schermer, the analyst's language and expressiveness must reach the analysand's body, "moving" it. "Emotions are *embodied* thoughts. Words and thoughts have bodily connotations: 'penetrating', 'hard', etc. The analyst's interpretations are emanations from his body that penetrate the patient's body. All of this harks back to childhood fantasies ..."[109]

* * *

This brings to a close the torrent of vignettes offered to the reader, with the expectation that this chapter is fulfilling its function of compiling psychoanalytical material that is extremely difficult for the Brazilian reader to access. This unprecedented compilation was the result of an extensive research effort, and this chapter is the most comprehensive undertaking possible at this moment, leaving for the future the possibility that this material may be reused and more thoroughly discussed, whether by myself or by another psychoanalyst colleague. Certainly, there are many positions that could be explored in their nuances.

To summarise, what can be pointed out is the clear disagreement between analysts as to the indication of the couch and its functions. However, I believe that we can (and should) see them as complementary. There is no doubt that all these positions enrich our discussion, and I take them all into account, even if implicitly, in what will be presented in Part II of this book.

Notes

1 Laplanche, (1987) 1993.
2 Laplanche, (1987) 1993, p. 150.
3 Laplanche, (1987) 1993, pp. 151–152.
4 Laplanche, (1987) 1993, p. 152.
5 Dejours, 2015.
6 Interview by Laplanche (2016), available at:www.bivipsi.org/wp-content/ uploads/percurso-2016-56-57-19.pdf.
7 Interview with Jacques André (2009), available at: psic.bvsalud.org/scielo.php?script=sci_arttext&pid=S0103-58352009000200002.
8 Accessed April 2021: wiberation.fr/cahier-special/1999/07/03/le-couch-xx1-e-siecle-demain-la-mondialisation-des-couchs-vers-le-corps-portable-par-jacques-alain-m_278498/?outputType=amp.
9 Cassullo, 2016, pp. 18–34.
10 Schmideberg, 1948, pp. 309–311.
11 Fenichel, (1941) 1961, pp. 44–46.
12 Fenichel, (1941) 1961.
13 Balint, 1959.
14 Balint, 1959, p. 95.
15 Abraham, 1942a.
16 Abraham, 1942b, p. 117.
17 Abraham, 1942, p. 189.
18 Rank, 2016.
19 Stern, 1945.
20 Stern, 1945, p. 193.
21 Stern, 1945, p. 198.
22 Eisenstein, 1951, pp. 379–401.
23 Eisenstein, 1951, p. 181.
24 Eisenstein, 1951, p. 192.
25 To this end, Eisenstein relies on this statement from Federn: "The most important self-defence against schizophrenia is neurosis, which is usually of the hysterical or obsessive type. No latent schizophrenic should be 'freed' from his neurosis, and he should definitely not be treated by the standard form of psychoanalysis." (Federn, 1947, pp. 129–145.)

26 Adler, 1988, pp. 353–372.
27 Santos and Mello Neto, 2018, pp. 285–293. Lable et al., 2010, pp. 861–887.
28 Ferro, 2009, p. 215.
29 The book that contains this account was written with Giuseppe Civitarese. The authors justify that, because they agree with all the positions shared in the publication, they sign the book entirely. They don't make it exactly clear, therefore, whether the case reported is in fact Ferro's or Civitarese's. In any case, both would agree, in technical terms, with what is reported in that chapter (Civitarese and Ferro, 2022, p. 6).
30 Sadow, 1995, pp. 386–395.
31 Kris, 1996.
32 Wolf, 1995, pp. 314–323.
33 Quinodoz, 2003.
34 Quinodoz, 2003, p. 1.476.
35 Quinodoz, 2003, pp. 1.479–1.480.
36 Quinodoz, 2003.
37 Deutsch, 1952, pp. 196–214.
38 Deutsch, 1952, p. 197.
39 McLaughlin, 1992, pp. 131–162.
40 Meltzer, (1984) 2009, p. 128.
41 Meltzer, 1992a pp. 102–103.
42 Meltzer, (1967) 2018; Meltzer and Harris, 2011; Meltzer, (1992b) 2008; Meltzer, 1994; Mélega, 2014.
43 Meltzer, (1992b) 2008, p. 23.
44 Bruni, 2013.
45 Bruni, 2013, p. 207.
46 Bruni, 2013, p. 211.
47 Staehle, 2013, p. 207.
48 Staehle, 2013, p. 207.
49 Durban, 2017.
50 The authors' clinical reports can be found in Mitrani and Mitrani, 2015.
51 Tustin, 1986, 1995.
52 See S. Klein, 2015 (*Autistic Phenomena in Neurotic Patients*), Houzel, 2015 (*Precipitation Anxiety in the Analysis of Adult Patients*) and J. Mitrani (*Trying to Enter the Long Black Branches: Some Technical Extensions for the Analysis of Autistic States in Adults*) in Mitrani and Mitrani, 2015.
53 Mitrani, 2015, p. 179.
54 Segal, (1956) 1981.
55 Segal, (1950) 1981.
56 Segal, (1950) 1981, p. 110.
57 Baudry, 2018.
58 Baudry, 2018, p. 185.
59 Eekhoff, 2017.
60 Eekhoff, 2017, p. 11.
61 Judy Eekhoff recounts the case in great detail, also presenting her theoretical and clinical reasoning in much more depth than here, which makes it impossible to exemplify without going into her case at length. The important thing here would be to point to a serious, life-threatening case that was thoroughly and successfully dealt with on the couch.
62 Eshel, 2017.
63 Korbivcher, 2017.
64 Korbivcher, 2017, p. 161.
65 Kelmon, 1954.
66 Jacobson, 1995.

67 Gedo, 1995, pp. 294–303.
68 Goldberger, 1995, pp. 23–42.
69 Skolnick, 2015, pp. 624–648.
70 Fairbairn, 1958, pp. 374–385.
71 Fairbairn, 1957.
72 Fairbairn, 1957, pp. 59–60.
73 Among them: Lable et al., 2010; Friedberg et al., 2012; Schachter and Kächele, 2010; Milton, 2003; Celenza, 2005.
74 Isaacs, (1952) 2002, p. 76.
75 Searles, 1960, p. 297.
76 Waugaman, 1995, p. 353. See also Searles, 1976.
77 Waugaman, 1995, p. 354.
78 Waugaman, 1995, pp. 338–357.
79 Waugaman, 1995, p. 338.
80 See Part I, Chapter 3, "The couch-body of Donald Woods Winnicott".
81 Waugaman, 1995, p. 341.
82 Guntrip, (1961) 1964, p. 391.
83 Guntrip, 1969.
84 Waugaman, 1995, p. 343.
85 Gabbard, 1991.
86 Waugaman, 1995, p. 349.
87 Rose, 1962.
88 Flournoy, 1979.
89 Waugaman, 1995, pp. 349, 352.
90 Hopkins, 2008.
91 Khan, 1996.
92 Hopkins, 2008, p. 273.
93 Hopkins, 2008, p. 80.
94 Hopkins, 2008, p. 153.
95 Hopkins, 2008, p. 203.
96 Hopkins, 2008, p. 266.
97 Hopkins, 2008, p. 268.
98 Lewin, 1955.
99 Lewin, 1955, p. 172.
100 Lewin, 1955, p. 190.
101 Lewin, 1955, p. 191.
102 Eissler, 1951.
103 Macalpine, 1950.
104 Macalpine, 1950, p. 522.
105 Heimann, (1958) 2005; (1975a) 2005a.
106 Heimann, (1975b) 2005.
107 Botella and Botella, 2005, p. 130.
108 Schermer, 2014.
109 Schermer, 2014, p. 180.

Chapter 15

Brief final comments

As becomes evident, although the title and content of the chapters in this first part of the book are intended to elucidate the clinical and theoretical positions of specific authors, these chapters are not just about that. The effort to problematise their contributions from a "textual listening" point of view has meant that, although these chapters are based on the authors' contributions, they are related to my particular reading of them, always trying to compare them with the chapters prior to their presentation and, obviously, leaving some of my positions on these contributions more latent or more explicit. Many of these I will not revisit directly in Part II, precisely because I have already made them explicit in the preceding chapters.

So, for those readers who may have skipped a chapter up to this point, I'd advise you to pick it up again, as they are all interconnected in one big discussion. My reservation is that, despite including my positions in these chapters, I have refrained from relating them to the basic conceptual terminology that underpins the second (more authorial) part of the book. I did this in order not to confuse or complicate the reader's understanding. Therefore, for a complete understanding of my position on the functions of the couch, although influenced by all these authors, Part II of the book is essential.

Any and all of my positions so far will be less complete if we don't take into account what follows, since these chapters in Part I have been marked by a terminological and theoretical abstinence from what is to come.

DOI: 10.4324/9781003681212-17

PART II

The poetics of psychoanalysis

Chapter 16

Introduction

An analyst's theoretical and clinical practice in dialogue with others

We've arrived here after listing and problematising various ways of thinking about the use of the couch. It's not a matter of agreeing or disagreeing, in whole or in part, with the reflections proposed by fellow psychoanalysts. Rather, it is about highlighting the diversity of listening and ways of conceiving the clinical device that we have used as psychoanalysts since the early days. I align myself with Christopher Bollas's view when he states that the (diverse) psychoanalytic theories are internal objects that we access when they are needed: in clinical practice. Therefore, I believe that all the points of view presented in Part I can be accessed by any analyst in the course of their work. It would be wrong to opt for a single path, to cling to just one understanding and blind oneself to complexity. The psychoanalytic movement cannot (or should not) function in a religious way, otherwise we will make standardised, sterile and even taboo-laden decisions.

Psychoanalysis has lost a lot and continues to lose a lot when groups of psychoanalysts close in around schools, around an author, around their own institutions, repeating a single thought. Therefore, I believe it is essential to listen to, study and dialogue with the diverse proposals of fellow psychoanalysts to find a place for them in our own theoretical-clinical practice. Otherwise, we would be replicating the famous couch of Procrustes,[1] bringing a dogmatic point of view to our clinic, without realising every nuance and variable involved in the couch, its use and, of course, the uniqueness of each human being we are listening to and working with. For this reason, authors who often "don't talk to each other" have been placed side by side in the same book. I believe that a good place to start this dialogue is on the couch.

In this second part of the book, I will rehearse the proposal of conceiving the couch and clinical practice through the metaphor *of* the *cloud state*. My intention is to share what has helped me in my work, as a kind of clinical listening model, which would complement (rather than replace) the rich propositions of the authors presented in Part I. It is my intention that the following proposals be received as an exchange of theoretical and clinical thoughts among colleagues. There is no staunch defence for what will be presented. My

DOI: 10.4324/9781003681212-19

intention is to continue offering new angles for listening beyond those already discussed in Part I.

When a poet writes about love, he is not reinventing it, but approaching it through a new *form*. He doesn't want to re-create love, re-invent love. The poet knows that love has been written about for millennia; his intention is simply to exercise a new *form* of enunciating it in his own way. When thinking about clinical practice, this proposition will have this horizon.

I'll start with an aspect that no psychoanalyst mentioned above in Part I has dealt with: the etymology of *couch/divan/diwan*. It's strange that this facet hasn't been explored before, given its enormous richness. After the etymology, which will serve as a trigger for the reflections that follow, I invite the reader to take a stroll through Goethe's "cloud play" and some other poetic influences, followed by additions involving play and *re-formation*, discussed in the light of fundamental concepts – such as *Verdichtung* (condensation), *Darstellung* (presentation), *symbolic vesture*, among some auxiliary constructs, such as *psychic regions*. Obviously, the proposal I put forward stems from a way of thinking that involves psychoanalytic clinical practice and the process of listening – including listening to children. The order of presenting these ideas, among other important considerations, **to weave the concept of the *couch/diwan* in a *cloud state***, has been redone and reordered countless times in an attempt to make the exposition as simple as possible. Given the range of facets addressed and the way the propositions articulate with one another, it is a fact that, in each chapter, there will always remain gaps to be worked through and rearticulated in subsequent chapters. Therefore, I ask the reader for patience in the hope that, in some way, at least part of what I essay below can be an element to contribute to their theoretical-clinical thinking. The exercise of *form* is always incomplete, it is always an attempt, but it seems essential to me that every analyst tries to develop one and share it with colleagues, even to rethink it.

Psychic life is essentially characterised by an eternal *re-forming*. When it comes to theoretical production, *re-forming* is also what Freud did throughout his work. What follows is my shared psychoanalytic theoretical-clinical exercise.

Note

1 Maud Mannoni (1991) tells us about the Greek legend of Procrustes, who offered travellers an iron bed to rest on that was his exact size. This supposedly generous gesture, however, was a trap: Procrustes placed his victims in the bed, moulding them according to the size of the bed (the exact size of Procrustes). Thus, if the victim was small, his body would be brutally stretched out; if the victim was larger than the bed, his parts would be amputated.

Chapter 17

Some considerations on the history and etymology of the word couch/*divan*/*diwan*

***Editorial note*: Before going further, the anglophone reader may wish to consult the initial note in this book's preliminary pages, "On the couch/*divã*/*divan*/*diván*/*diwan*: key considerations regarding the English edition", for a better understanding of the terms evoked here and their interconnections.**

Why, only at this point in the book, do I bring up the etymology? This is the first time that a psychoanalytic theoretical-clinical proposal has used the etymology of the couch to think about its use. It wouldn't make sense to present the etymology before presenting the thoughts of all the authors present in the first part, since none of them takes the etymology as a reference for thinking about clinical practice, nor mentions it.

"*Diwan*" is a Persian term for writer or scribe. Later, it came to signify a collection – a gathered work – of poems, usually by a single author, produced from the 7th century onward. Goethe, for example, one of the *Dichter*[1] most admired by Freud, published in 1819 the book *West-östlicher Divan*[2] (*West–Eastern Divan*), inspired by the *Diwan of Hāfez*,[3] read by Muslims as a book of wisdom (alongside the Qur'an).

Although poetics has been central to Freud and to psychoanalysis from the very beginning, the nomenclature of the piece of furniture he eventually adopted in his clinical practice seems to derive from other branches. The Arabic branch of *diwan* also alludes to registry, cabinet or administration. This terminology is still used for government spaces and positions in various countries in the Middle East and Asia. In a Turkish-Ottoman context, the term referred to the very council of state itself or the Sultan's meeting room. Historically, the Turks had private audience rooms, the council of the sultans, filled with cushions (a kind of sofa without armrests or backrests). The modern word "*aduana*", customs, which is a government office that controls the entry and exit of goods (and people) from one territory to another, and where taxes are also levied, is also derived from *diwan*.

So then … why bring up such matters here?

It is only by starting from these expositions that we can begin to think about the many aspects of the couch's use in the analytic room. Let us take the

DOI: 10.4324/9781003681212-20

exercise of following the associative play that etymology offers us. First, the term *diwan* (couch) contains within it (from its ancestral reminiscences)[4] a notion of space. A space in which, among other functions, a body rests. I repeat, not only is the furniture a space where a body rests, but also the word itself. And it's not just any space: it's a meeting space of the utmost importance. A powerful space? What kind power? What kind of state? Under what laws? An oppressive space (it can be, if used inappropriately)? Or a space for creating a better (internal) world? A space for experiential exchange? These and countless other more complex questions could be asked about this space.

From its origin, as we have just seen, the *divan* (*couch*) also points us to a space of records. Thus, we can think of the couch as a space that contains, holds and moves records. If the couch is a space that contains records, we begin to get closer to Freudian metapsychology: Is the couch itself an "incarnation"[5] of the Unconscious in a piece of furniture? Or is the couch a customs house (*aduana*)? A space of transition, or regulation, between what comes in and what goes out? A space where, from an economic point of view, agreements are made and taxes paid? Is the couch the place where compromises have to be made? Is it where economic negotiations take place about what can leave and what should stay (through speech/declarations)? There are those who try to dodge customs, to hide their belongings when they pass through, just like the disguise employed in the return of the repressed. All these facets are contained in the function of the couch. It's *as if* the couch could be the "incarnation" of the Unconscious, and even of compromise formation.

Let's also reflect on the poetic prism that this etymology offers us. The *couch/divan/diwan* as a scribe, a recorder – the couch (and those who lie on it) as a writer. It's not easy to write a book. Writing, revising, rewriting, repeating these three steps again and again. How do you construct, deconstruct and reconstruct the text? How does one carry out this aesthetic labour? The couch as collection of poems is a very powerful image. Being the space that contains the book of scriptures, the collected works of an author, is something of the most intimate relic. Are we looking at a new book to be written? A re-edition to be revised? A battered edition with torn pages? Blank pages? Erasures? Stains? Some touching poems? Poems still in the making? Beauties yet to be explored? Or the misery of enunciation?

Every poem has a formal structure, whether it belongs to the so-called "fixed forms" or to free verse. Each poem has its own rhythm, its unique combinations of words. Poetry also has its schools, its theories, its angles, its choices. Why is one word placed next to another? Which poems do we like, and which do we not? Which poems seem to lack strength, and which poems make us feel? Which poem touches us? How can we write our lives better? Or, still, how can we accept ourselves, even if we are not such good poets?

The poem contains gaps, words placed upon the whiteness of the page. Within each word and in the blank spaces between them lies an immense creative potential. And here we return to the question of space – the couch/diwan as an "incarnation" of the analysand's Unconscious, as a transitional space between the analytic pair, and, above all, as a third space that enables the unfolding of psychoanalytic work. Whatever the perspective, it is undoubtedly a potential space. We cannot deny that the psychoanalytic couch bears within itself the potency of the *diwan* in its full amplitude, and that, upon it, psychic life is projected.

Notes

1 Next, we'll work in more depth on *Dichter*, a word more usually translated as poet, but which has a slightly broader dimension.
2 Goethe, (1819) 2020.
3 Hāfez or Hafiz was a Persian lyricist and mystic, born between 1310 and 1337. See Hafez, 2019.
4 Part I, Chapter 1, "Sigmund Freud's couch-reminiscence", discussed looking at the use of the couch from the perspective of reminiscence.
5 The term isn't quite right, I know … furniture doesn't have flesh on it, but I think that's the best name for it.

Chapter 18

Play as the essence of the psychoanalytic process

18.1 Freud's child poet and Goethe's cloud play

"Great elephant! Stretch out your trunk,"
says the child to the stretching cloud.
And the cloud obeys.

Ludwig Tieck (1773–1853)[1]

If it's useful to think of the couch from its etymology, let's continue in this vein. Let's not forget to take into account what has been seen etymologically as a "space for important meetings" and its customs-like function, among other issues previously raised, but I will begin by developing my thought from the poetic etymology of the couch/diwan. It's nothing new for readers of Freud to see how poetic art runs through his work and helps him construct his theory. In a large part of his writings, we find poetic-literary quotations, such as, for example, the numerous passages from Goethe's *Faust*, present in the *The Interpretation of Dreams*,[2] which we will return to when presenting the theoretical proposal of *symbolic vesture* and *psychic weaving*.

More than Freud's poetic quotes, we are mainly interested in what he says about the creational/creative process. I use the term *creational* because it is richer than it seems. The basis of creationism is that there is a god who creates the world, and if we're talking about the child who creates its world omnipotently, we're talking about the *creational*,[3] that is, the act of generating/creating a world in and of itself. The baby is even more than "his majesty", as Freud pointed out in *Introduction to Narcissism*;[4] he is a kind of creator-god,[5] who works on the fine line between creating his psychic reality and apprehending the world around him. In the essay *Der Dichter und das Phantasieren*[6] – which has many translation options,[7] including "the poet[[8]] and fantasising", we have the statements that "in every man hides a poet" and that "every child who plays behaves like a poet, since he creates his own world for himself". For Freud, "the poet does the same as the child who plays".[9] Thus, if we combine the propositions of the founder of psychoanalysis with Winnicott's play, we can

DOI: 10.4324/9781003681212-21

say that children play at building worlds, and it is in this way that they build/write and poeticise their own world. Artistic creation depends on the ability to access *the child that lives within*, and so does the psychoanalytic process.

It's remarkable that Freud's positions are similar to the poetic realm of the *couch/diwan*. It is also a historical fact that Freud used to cover his couch with Persian rugs: was this pure coincidence? Freud didn't believe in coincidence; he believed that the Unconscious determined choices. Could covering his couch with one of the greatest symbols of Persian culture be seen as reinforcing the presence of poetry, alluding to the Persian etymology of *diwan*, in his theoretical-clinical work? Regardless of the answer, I imagine that Freud probably did not think of this consciously, yet would have found such speculations at least interesting and amusing. I am speaking here of play, and psychic health depends on play. In psychoanalysis, what matters more is preserving the possibility of the coexistence of *multiple internal truths* rather than remaining fixed upon a single conclusion – a simplification of the vast world that exists within each human being.

The central point that unites childhood, the poet and the work on the couch, which I intend to elucidate, involves the evocation of internal processes of transformation. When I published simultaneously my book of poems *Homage to the Cloud* (2017)[10] and the collection of essays *Interlocutions on the Border Between Psychoanalysis and Art* (2017),[11] I was led, internally and naturally, to unite/condense my speech around foundational concepts that resonated across these two works. Gradually, I began to develop a kind of transposition of the poetic conceptuality explored in *Homage to the Cloud* – the conceptuality of "cloud" that I was working with aesthetically – into a possible metaphor for psychoanalytic work, particularly with regard to the *couch/diwan*. This metaphor eventually culminated in the writing of the present book, since it came to accompany me throughout the process of listening in the analytic setting from that point onward.

Conceiving the session and the couch/*diwan* as *a cloud state* – and as part of a "cloud play" – may serve as a valuable facilitator when working with the language of childhood[12] that emerges in the analytic process. It seems to me that this proposal would be helpful in psychoanalytic processes with analysands who had a "good enough" childhood, but also with those who didn't have such an opportunity, if we think that one of the functions of play is also to elaborate the traumatic. As was seen in the first part of the book and as will be discussed below, psychoanalytic listening and intervention from the couch can be broader than the classic model proposes.

It is essential that an analysis also includes the exercise of creative pleasure. To relinquish a neurosis or symptom, one must be convinced that, in giving up the infantile that binds (while still offering secondary gains), one is not abandoning the childhood that lives within – the ludic capacity – which, on the contrary, is what brings liberation. For fear that analysis might extinguish their creativity, many talented artists, burdened with intense suffering, avoided it – as Ferenczi already pointed out in 1928.[13] Play cannot be absent from any process of analysis, whether in those who retain internal traces (from childhood) of creative play, or in those who must first come into contact with this modality of relating to the world. To reawaken the capacity to play with life – or, depending on the case, to bring it into existence for the first time – is integral to the process of analysis.

The incessant movement of clouds may serve as an interesting metaphor for thinking about psychic work on the couch, and this proposal is closely linked to what would be the order of *creational processes*. I invite the reader to the development of this idea, beginning with a small yet fruitful fragment from the work of Goethe, who exercised great influence on Freud and served as a source of theoretical inspiration.

Although his literary fame is greater, Goethe was very involved with his scientific side. His studies of natural sciences included anatomy, osteology, botany, nephology (the study of clouds) and meteorology, as well as chemistry, geology, mineralogy and zoology. Goethe even wrote a "cloud diary"[14] and devoted himself intensely to these studies, working directly with the meteorological instruments available in his time. "The observation of clouds in Goethe always has an *empirical* and a *symbolic* side"[15] writes Portuguese translator João Barrento.

In 1817, when he set out to briefly explain and exemplify the work of Luke Howard (the father of modern meteorology), Goethe named a technical essay on clouds *Camarupa*, "the name of an Indian deity who enjoys changing forms".[16] In this text, he also emphasised the "playfulness of clouds", in his own words: an acknowledgment that Goethe brought scientific thought, discovery and the development of a science into alignment with the act of play, rendering them inseparable. He invested in clouds both their scientific and ludic potential at once. This suggests that even science and scientists require the playfulness of art and play itself in order to advance.

This perspective of Goethe, which permeates the paradox of the meteorological truth of clouds and their ludic play, will serve as a guide for the path to be followed from this point onward. The ideas that clouds[17] can carry a latent truth (a "something more") that can be accessed from their forms, and that there is "play" in them,[18] are intrinsically linked to the proposal I intend to bring into the discussion.

18.2 The clouds, the poets and Vicente Huidobro's creationism

Let's continue our reflection on the clouds, leaving the theme of the *couch/diwan* in latency at this point, as conceptualised by Roussillon.[19] The poet Murilo Mendes, loved and admired by European avant-garde artists, who quoted Freud a lot and whose work is explicitly influenced by Freud's concepts of the Unconscious and sexuality, can help us. Murilo Mendes was a professor of literature in Rome and is one of the most important voices in Brazilian poetry, although he is currently less well known to the general public than he should be. His debut book, *Poemas* (1930),[20] won the most important award in the country, surpassing, for example, Carlos Drummond de Andrade's first book. A friend and collaborator of the surrealist movement idealised by André Breton, Murilo Mendes preferred to see himself "outside" the movement, believing in the singularity of thought and poetry as the path against totalitarianism of thought (common to any kind of avant-garde at the time).

From his vast body of work, I would like to highlight how Mendes uses clouds as the raw material for profound communication – clouds that, aesthetically, serve to unsettle and create new perspectives. There is a fundamental morphological point contained in them that perhaps nothing else on our planet resembles. In the work of Murilo Mendes, we find countless allusions to clouds, but they are central figures in the book *Metamorphoses* (1944).[21] "The seas contract / the clouds stretch their wings" – the poet points to the expansion and liberation of flight. "The wandering cloud welcomes the bird / That has left the stone statue / I am that wandering cloud, / The bird and the stone statue" – alludes to the paradox. "Yes: letter and cloud / fight with dreams / For possession of the poem" – accuses the conflict. "Anonymous clouds: seek my thirst" –summons desire.

The verses quoted here are just a third of how clouds are presented in the book. In Murilo Mendes' poetic work, mentions of clouds also serve to elucidate war and destruction; and they do not leave out his look at social helplessness: "ancient cloud, you are the beginning of the dance, / the construction of reality, the poetry of the poor...", or, let's be fair, his verse would allude to much more than that. The cloud is democratic and it's for everyone. It is the object of play that everyone can access; but it is more, because poetry is and goes beyond what theoretical prose can try to describe.

The cloud is paradoxical from every angle from which we can analyse it. Firstly, it is part of the condemned play of any "successful" childhood. And, unlike expensive and/or electronic toys, it is accessible to every child, regardless of socioeconomic background. In general, every child has at least access to the cloud (or its *Darstellung* function).[22] It may be seen as the playful lifeline of an otherwise arid life.

In *Dream and Myth: A Study in the Psychology of Peoples*,[23] Karl Abraham works with various myths – including religious ones – to demonstrate how "the heavens" and their phenomena served as a "place" for transposing the infantile and unconscious psychic phenomena of peoples. In this sense, we could briefly state that, since the very beginnings of humanity, through displacement, condensation and compromise formations, human beings have projected onto the skies, the sun, the moon, and the clouds what truly belonged to their internal and unconscious realm.

Clouds have always accompanied poets (creators). There would be too little space in this book if we wanted to list all the beautiful verses that project aspects of psychic life on to the clouds.[24]

Playing/working psychically with the phenomena of nature is what all ancient peoples have always done. All myths are built upon this play. Nature is the primal material of mythological, religious and cultural constructions. "Myth originates from an ancestral period in the life of a collective of people, which we can designate as the childhood of the people,"[25] says Karl Abraham. The cloud is the most malleable and transformational representative of this childhood play, and I would venture to say that the cloud is one of humanity's oldest "toys" – if not the oldest.

From the perspective of primary narcissistic omnipotence, seeing a horse in a cloud does not raise the question of whether it was the child who observed it or the cloud that offered such a figure. *Creational* omnipotence[26] is essential for a child's healthy development. As Winnicott advocates, this experience needs to be lived and not explained. It's not a question of differentiating whether the child created an object or whether it was given to them by someone else. This omnipotence is narcissising, strengthens the *self* and guarantees confidence in future movements. The same premise would apply to a traumatic childhood experience. Not being able to experience this omnipotence would, at the very least, lead to a lack of confidence in oneself and the risk of developing narcissistic pathologies.[27]

The Chilean poet Vicente Huidobro, an avant-gardist of creationism – a revolutionary poetic movement that influences other movements, such as the surrealist and the concretist – is the author of the verse "The Poet is a Little God".[28] In this, it is *as if* Huidobro translated Freud and condensed Freud's theorization of infantile omnipotence, linking it to the creative act. Such questions should not be taken as language embellishments.

When psychoanalysts set out to work with the infantile, and this is a premise of our discipline, they must also work with the omnipotent character of "primitive" psychic functioning allied with creativity. Let us take omnipotence here in the sense of creating a world, creating oneself and one's internalities. The analysand lying on the couch *has created (and is constantly creating) the world in which he lives.* We need to access it, but, more than that, we need to experience this world in the session.

18.3 The *diwan* as cloud – re-form in analysis

The space of the session, the *diwan*, as a spatiality, in its condition as a space for important meetings, as we have seen from the etymology, is a potential space to be psychically re-actualised from the virtuality of the transference[29] and the atmosphere of the session. The analysand's internal world is transposed into the analytic room and onto all the elements that compose it, while the analyst is summoned to occupy transferential roles within a plot proposed by this internal world.

The psychoanalytic process unfolds from the role that the analyst will play in the analysand's internal world, actualised in session, into which the analyst is naturally "pulled into". Any technical move by the analyst is an intervention in this world that he or she has been summoned to inhabit. Their role involves questioning the geography and architecture of the analysand's internal constructions and perhaps, through their psychic apparatus, offering new materials for their constructions. How the analysand makes use of these "materials" offered by the psychoanalyst is their own prerogative; however, the analyst accompanies him in this internal updating, either questioning what has been built (how it was built and why it was) or offering new materials for it. In any psychoanalytic work, the analyst is an object that aids an internal *re-formation.*

So, at this point in our discussion, it doesn't matter so much whether we're talking about levels of suffering or psychopathological types, but rather that the psychoanalyst's role is always to help *re-form* the internal world of their analysands. The process of analysis aims to create and re-create forms and, although it involves the analyst, it is a process of the analysand – the creator (and re-creator) of himself. The analytic process is a process of *re-forming* oneself, of offering new ways of seeing and of living with oneself.

An analysis works insofar as it deals with the internal processes that are necessary to make a story multiple stories (to live together in new versions) – in other words, to explore the multiple that lives within oneself, as will be further elaborated with regard to the *psychic regions*. We can never entirely erase a former version of ourselves; all that is left is to learn how to coexist with it, for it remains alive within us until our final breath, even when we try to turn away from it (and deny it any possibility of dialogue).

In this sense, we could say that the ultimate psychoanalytical aim would be to *re-form*: to work from the internal processes that create forms. To *re-form* would be the exact opposite of the deadly repetition compulsion. Instead of repeating the same form, there would be a "repetition" of the act of creating new forms. After all, I don't think we can escape the prefix "re" in psychic life. If we think from the point of view of health, the best thing we can do would be to "repeat" the act of *re-forming*, of finding various vertices to understand and cohabit with each other – integrate – because the aim is not to find an internal truth, but rather to acknowledge sometimes paradoxical internal truths, which oppose one another and are not necessarily correlated.

For example: the "truth" of the Freudian first topic is different from the second. In some respects, the psychic apparatuses proposed by Freud resemble one another; in others, they diverge. The functioning of one topic is no more "true" than that of the other, nor has the creation of the second made the first "die". It's *as if* these two "theoretical worlds" could inhabit the same human being. However, beyond this theoretical and dualistic example, we might then think of an infinity of "versions" of ourself coexisting internally within each human being – even if some may be more mortified, while others are yet to be born.

To *re-form* ("to create forms") would thus be the counterpoint to the deadly compulsion to repeat, based on ways relating to oneself and the world. Playing is

re-forming*. In this sense, we could think of the work on the *couch/diwan* as a cloud – in its capacity to generate forms. Following the reflections of the authors we have seen earlier, the couch would be a kind of couch-cloud-body-womb-mother-analyst that serves as a support for the processes of forming and *reforming*. In this way, we would be thinking of psychoanalytic work in *a cloud state[30] – propositions that need to be further developed in subsequent chapters, to avoid the risk of them being understood as simplistic or careless.

Notes

1 Author's version.
2 Freud, 1900.
3 Later on, we'll return to the term *creational*, based on the Chilean poet Vicente Huidobro.
4 Freud, (1914a) 1996f.
5 This idea will be discussed more clearly a few pages below.
6 Freud, 1908a [1907] 2015a.
7 Some of these options are: *Creative Writers and Daydreams*, *The Poet and the Fan* and *The Writer and Fantasy* (2015), with Brazilian translations from 2006 (published by Imago), 2014 (published by Hedra) and 2015b (published by Companhia das Letras), respectively.
8 Creative writer, as *Dichter* was translated in Freud's *Obras completas*, published by Imago (2006), is also linked to the Persian etymology of *couch/diwan*, see above.
9 Freud, (1908b [1907]) 2014.
10 Krüger, 2017c.
11 Krüger, 2017 contains the essay "Poetry, Listening and the Use of Words in the Psychoanalytic Clinic", an initial sketch on the subject.
12 Ferenczi's term.
13 Ferenczi, (1928), 1992.
14 This and other material by Goethe on meteorology and clouds are compiled in the book *The Cloud Play* (2003).
15 Barrento, 2003.
16 Goethe, 2003.
17 I'm already thinking about the metaphorical character I intend to develop.
18 This proposal is closely linked to Ferenczi's work analysing through play and welcoming the child who lives in the adult. See Part I, Chapter 2, "The couch, the child who lives in the adult, and the technical daring of Sándor Ferenczi".
19 See Part I, Chapter 9, "René Roussillon's couch in latency".
20 Mendes, (1930) 2014.
21 Mendes, (1944) 2015.
22 The concept of *Darstellung* will be presented in more detail in a later chapter.
23 Abraham, (1909) 2020.
24 *Editor's note*: In the present edition, this passage has been abridged. In the original publication, it was followed by an extensive selection of verses from various authors, in which 'the clouds' assumed a prominent role.
25 Abraham, (1909), 2020.
26 A term that we began to contextualise in Section 18.1 "Freud's child-poet and Goethe's cloud play".
27 I ask the reader not to stick firmly to conflicting theoretical terms that may appear throughout the text. One reader may prefer to "listen" to this text from the

perspective of the narcissism coined by Freud, while another, from the perspective of the development of the *self* in Winnicott. I don't think we should exclude these understandings. Let's live with the theoretical paradox and the overlapping of terms, which lead us to different understandings of psychic functioning. As the theoretical proposal of this book is more to open up a range of potential listenings than to defend a univocal idea, the paradox of enunciation becomes more important than a supposed "limpid clarity" that would close doors to different forms of interpretation.

28 Poem originally in the book *El espejo de agua* (Huidobro, 1916).

29 After all, virtuality is an intrinsic characteristic of the transference – for example, the analysand relating to the analyst *as if* they were the father, *as if* they were the mother, etc.

30 Based on its character as "the creation of forms", what has been presented before, and what will be presented next.

Chapter 19

The psychic regions and the cloud state

Human beings are always on the move and have a tendency to create from the moment they begin to create themselves, even if this depends on another person. Creation is always based on a relationship, but it would be too naïve to think theoretically of total passivity in the creation of the psyche. Freud[1] theorises and emphasises repetition from a symptomatic perspective, but not only that: his theoretical models demonstrate that the psyche is a *creational* engine. If, on the one hand, the symptom is repetition, on the other, it is the product of the psychic *creational* process. So we can't confuse creation with psychic health either. We also create psychic mechanisms that end up causing us suffering.

At this point, I propose approaching the *creational* from the *cloud state* perspective.[2] However, as was the case in the previous chapters, some of the proposals in this chapter will require further elaboration regarding the concepts of *Darstellung* (presentation), *Ditchtung* (poetry), *Verdichtung* (condensation) and *symbolic vesture*, which will be considered next.

All the psychic resources of each singular human being are susceptible to activation, whenever it is possible to work from what I am calling the *cloud state* – within the psychoanalytic session. On the one hand, if we follow a psychic model predominantly based on the first Freudian topic, the *cloud state* could be seen as the deepest and most primitive movement of psychic regression/regredience.[3] However, such an affirmation would be incomplete, for this line of thought would lead us only to what belongs to the order of the primitive processes and defence mechanisms of the psyche. The *cloud state* proposal is a little different, because it presupposes a *state*. Let me explain.

There are at least two ways of looking at the notion of *state*. In the case of the cloud, let's start by thinking about the state of water. The cloud is a form of the water's *presentification*, a way for water to *present itself*. The cloud is a cluster of minuscule particles – of liquid water or ice (or both) – suspended in the atmosphere, along with particles from, for example, industrial vapours and smoke (which would open the way for us to think about *pollution from the outside having an impact on the inside* – "Does smoke talk to clouds?" Pablo Neruda (1974) would ask in his verses). For this example, it's not even

DOI: 10.4324/9781003681212-22

necessary to go into chemical and physical formulations; let's just look at the "suspension" of the cloud, and think about the notion of state from a geographical territorial point of view:

The world is divided into continents, economic blocs, countries, states, cities, etc. We may divide/decompose the world from any angle we like. We have democratic states and totalitarian states. The world had been divided into countless colonies run by other nations, to a lesser or greater degree. Each country organizes itself politically in different ways – what they all have in common is territoriality. Borders determine the functioning of each regime, and we know, for example, that the laws in India are not the same as those in Brazil. With this metaphor, the intention is to point out that there are internal state-territories that function differently, often in conflict with one another. Could such a description be transposed to the functioning of the internal world?

André Green places psychoanalysts under the duty of advancing ever further into the "pieces of territory of the as yet unknown continent of the human mind".[4] Let's follow his proposal and ask: Does the human mind have just one continent? And if it has more, what would they be? We don't need to go into this "theoretical fiction" (to use the term coined by Freud[5] to describe his metapsychology), but it might be interesting to take the metaphor further.

From a certain point of view, the postulation of the Freudian concept of Superego/Supereu[6] could be an example of the creation of an internal region that has its own functioning. I don't intend to postulate more psychic regions, but I believe that we should think that each psyche has countless of them, each with micro-functions – and perhaps not always with similar "cultures", if compared to the psyche of others. Let's think of the Superego as a continent; within it, there are different countries, with different states, different cities, different political groups fighting for power in each of these regions … Moreover, the term "Superego", originally coined by Freud, has been subjected to countless theoretical variations by other authors.

If we want to opt for another way of classifying these regions, we could think of them as psychic mechanisms intrinsically linked to certain pathologies. Bion[7] proposes a psychic model in which there are overlapping areas. For him, a psychotic subject can have a non-psychotic part, just as a neurotic subject would also have a psychotic part. The emergence of one of these psychic regions would conceal the other, and, according to him, both must be analysed.

This idea of psychic areas/regions is explored by various authors in their own way. Green writes about an area of private madness;[8] Cassorla[9] mentions "more or less symbolic areas, psychotic areas, traumatic areas and areas without representation"; Bollas[10] writes about internal areas/states of creation, such as the *genera*, as well as the existence of a fascist state of mind, with a totalitarian functioning that would aim to dominate and/or destroy other regions;[11] Stefano Bolognini talks about desert regions;[12] while Marucco[13] proposes psychic zones, based on psychopathological structures that demonstrate, through clinical analysis, manifestations of zones that coexist and overlap simultaneously in the psychic apparatus. It would not be an arduous task to cite further examples here that corroborate a movement in contemporary psychoanalytic thinking towards a proposal for the coexistence of internal regions with different functions.

To begin reflecting on the diversity of internal functioning from the vantage point of clinical experience, let us borrow the words of Luís Claudio Figueiredo:

> Freud believed only in the neurotic transferences of the so-called "transference neuroses". It has been known for many decades that in addition to neurotic transferences, there are narcissistic, borderline, psychosomatic and psychotic transferences, all of which can participate in the formation of the analysing situation in its virtuality.[14]

What we know about history (of humanity and our planet) is that discoveries never cease. The use of oil, for example, is part of recent history. Brazil was "discovered" by the European world just over 500 years ago, even though life here is much older than that "discovery". It is a scientific fact that, even today, humanity continues to discover previously unknown species of animals and plants. Could it be that with 500 years of psychoanalysis, we're not thinking even more deeply and thoroughly about Freud's initial propositions?

So, how can we approach what has been thought regarding *cloud state*, including this notion of *psychic regions*? The clinical model I wish to propose is that the cloud is "suspended", hovering above all these internal states/regions. It feeds on the "climatic phenomena" of all these states: it requires the "water" that evaporates from them and "harvests" this water as fuel for forms, shadows and storms within each of these regions.

Psychoanalytic theories can be seen as state-regions, nothing more than "technological-theoretical" blocks (and fictional ones, as Freud himself points out) that serve as a kind of filter-lens to deal with the deep waters. Thus, the theories of various psychic apparatuses that we have are just the intermediary, the way of dealing with the deep water that is present in forms in the cloud. It's *as if* what is made *present* (in the sense of form) depends both on the raw matter (water-psi energy) and the "psychic-technological" resources of each region. A region with a psychotic mode of functioning will lend a psychotic character to the formation of the cloud.

I'm not proposing a new metapsychological model, nor am I trying to theoretically create or rearticulate structural psychic mechanisms based on this notion of psychic regions and the *cloud state*. Certainly, this model would be insufficient for this, but it seems adequate for the purpose of this book. However, it is possible to articulate this metaphor as a way of working, in the clinic, with the psychic regions that inhabit the analysand. After all, from the very beginning, this book has set out to describe various forms of listening – with the explicit aim of opening possibilities for working in psychoanalytic practice.

The *cloud state* is a state that triggers (in the sense of setting in motion) processes of undifferentiation between internal and external instances/regions, but this is not analogous to a regression. There are boundaries between internally delimited regions across which no passage is allowed. Exchange between internal regions only takes place to the extent that evaporated water "mixes" into the cloud. And it can travel through all the regions, offering new forms, rains and internal storms that can consequently affect and even modify the other psychic regions.

It is from this perspective that "the important meeting room" (*diwan*) works in a *cloud state*. Analytical work is with the derivatives of the inaccessible internal raw material. We can only access and possibly modify the internal regions of a psyche by working with "the clouds" that contain the derivatives of such matter (unconscious material). In analysis, we invariably work with what is *condensed* and *presented*. The psychoanalyst is called upon to take part in the plot that the analysand's *cloud* presents, occupying a transferential role that ends up "gaining" access to the contents and ways of functioning of their psychic regions.

Let's think of free association and floating attention as techniques that aim to act in the *cloud state*. On the one hand, *the cloud* is the space of the *Spiel/play*; on the other, it "gathers" material from the psychic regions. It is the surface contact between two psychic worlds.[15] **The basic proposal of the psychoanalytic technique is to move (float) over all the psychic regions, because what comes from these associations (from what is *presented* on the manifest level) is not the unconscious material itself. What we hear, in free association, is only a derivative – and it is in this light that we may think of the *cloud*: as the space in which the derivatives of the most varied psychic regions meet. From this perspective, the *cloud state* is a mobile/malleable territory of playing and also serves as a stage for compromise formations or other more disruptive *presentations*.**

To a certain extent, although I'm composing a different map here, the idea of working from the *cloud state* can be considered similar to what authors such as Fred Busch[16] and Stefano Bolognini[17] have said about working and intervening from the preconscious of the analysands. Their positions seem very sensible to me; after all, it's audacious to believe that we have the "power" to intervene directly in the unconscious of those being analysed, if not from the contents that are more on the surface. It is only through work with this material that we may, to some extent, aspire for unconscious contents to be touched.

Clouds form, but they also dissolve, returning the raw material (water) from which they drew in their formation. It is a virtual place of temporary storage, a transitory archive, like files that expire over time. The *cloud* is not static, in its essence, it is continually forming, re-forming, de-forming and dissolving, and this movement does not cease for a single second during the psychoanalytic session (or in life). Thus, in line with what has been said above, and as Luis Claudio Figueiredo would emphasise,[18] the clinical device and the transference are essentially virtual, regardless of whether the session is remote or face-to-face.

In the geography of each one's internal world, we can say that there are developed regions-states, "good technologies", "high investment capacity". Some have more unexplored and uninhabited inner deserts than others, while others live with a predominance of internal fascist states.[19] The internal world is as complex as the natural world. We all have regions with neurotic, psychotic, traumatic/arid, traumatic/polluted predominance. We have the pinnacle of civilisation and technology on the one hand, and, on the other, children (*internal potentials*) dying of hunger. The metaphor of the cloud is interesting if we think about it from the perspective that clouds can move and hover over all internal states. In every human being, there is a particular and unique internal planet.

The *cloud state* is neither the most primitive nor the most sublime. It's what hovers, transits and feeds back into every internal region, every internal functioning and every relationship with the external world. It's a multidimensional state that hovers over every other. And, of course, the *cloud of* each human being will depend how the psychic regions of each singular being function. This theoretical proposal will have to test its pertinence over the course of this writing.

Notes

1 Freud, (1914a) 2010.
2 A more poetic version of the reasoning that follows could rest on Mark Strand's line: "Every lake desires a cloud" (2016).
3 I use the two terms on purpose, even though they are not analogous, depending on the basis on which the reader is relying to understand the reasoning. At this point, neither term gets in the way of where I want us go.
4 Green, (1979a) 1988, p. 35.
5 Freud, (1900) 2019, p. 657.
6 Following this metaphor, we could think that within the Superego there are also micro-regions that interrelate. Within it, there would be censorious instances, linked to the interdictions, prohibitions, taboos and dikes described in the first Freudian topic; and, at the same time, instances linked to identities and ideals.
7 Bion, (1957) 1991.
8 Green, (1979b) 1988.
9 Cassorla, (2013) 2016, p. 42.
10 Bollas, (1992) 1998.
11 Krüger, 2021.
12 Bolognini, 2022, p. 192.
13 Marucco, 2003, 2012, 2013.
14 Figueiredo, 2020, p. 73.
15 André Green, when working on the notion of the border between the internal and the external, its surfaces and edges, evoking the notion of customs (the anus and the mouth as customs between the internal and the external), mentions a "state of intersection, a limit that resembles the meeting of two clouds" [Green, (1977) 1988, p. 69]. Although Green doesn't elaborate on the metaphor he has created, it certainly ties in with the metaphor we are discussing.

16 Busch, 2017.
17 Bolognini, 2022.
18 Figueiredo, 2020, pp. 61–80.
19 Christopher Bollas analyses the existence of an internal fascist region, which would seek to subjugate other psychic regions. See more on this in: Krüger, 2021; Bollas, 1998.

Chapter 20

The cloud, condensation and poetic creation

Reflections on *Dichter*, *Dichtung* and *Verdichtung*

The cloud helps us to dream transformation, Gaston Bachelard[1] teaches. Clouds are made up of droplets of condemned water. So we need to take a look at the Freudian conceptualisation *of Verdichtung/condensation* and, to do so, there is nothing is more appropriate than to decompose the word *Verdichtung*, so that we may glimpse what is itself condensed within it. I begin, therefore, by pointing out that the *Dichter*, the poet, is contained "within" condensation/*Verdichtung*. The verb *dichten* is intimately linked to the act of composing and, indeed, often connected to what we might call the "field of poetry". Haroldo de Campos[2] defines the word *Dichtung* (poetry, in its literal translation) as "verbal work of art", emphasising its essence as endowed with a "secret poeticity". Therefore, before seeking an equivalent for *Dichter* in Portuguese, it is essential to understand its essence. A *Dichter* is, above all, someone who makes a verbal work of art in which a secret poeticity resides. This idea is fundamental for thinking about the words spoken in session, whether by the analyst or the analysand.

Going further, *dicht* means dense; and *Verdichtung*/condensation is one of the most important terms in Freudian metapsychology. *Verdichtung* could also be translated as concentration, compression and compaction. Therefore, by following the avenues the word opens up, and already making a "condensation" (in Freudian terms), *Verdichtung* would present itself as a paradoxical term, for it indicates, at the same time, the compacting of something and the poet-making of that something. It is not by chance that Ezra Pound[3] presents the equation *Dichten = Condensare*, which we might freely translate as "to condense is to compose". In this way, when we refer to *Verdichtung* (condensation), it is important to take into account all these aspects of poetry and poetic-making that it carries.

Taking some distance from German, let's look at how Paul Valéry describes *poetics*, pointing to its etymology: "the name of everything related to the creation or composition of works in which language is both substance and medium – and not in the restricted sense of choosing rules or aesthetic precepts related to poetry".[4] His assertion is that the "poet" is not the one who makes poems,

DOI: 10.4324/9781003681212-23

just as poetics is not tied to poetry – which allows us to slide his explanation into what Freud proposes when relating poetic-making to childhood play.

Within the original Greek word *poiesis*, Valéry emphasises the making, *poiein*, the act of realising a work. "An expression originating from the verb *poiéo* (to make, to execute, to confect), *poiesis* translates as manufacture, confection, preparation, production."[5] There is a certain craftsmanship in giving form to what is, at first, only potential matter – which holds a latent potential depending on how it is handled. Yet the poet Percy Shelley refers to *poiein* as the "principle of synthesis".[6]

All the elements that I'm highlighting here lead us toward the psyche's inherent tendency to create, to combine, to condense, to synthesise. Let us listen to the words and their resonances: the cloud is a condensation; within the condensation/cloud there is the poet and the poetic act; and poetic-making itself is condensation.

Therefore, when I propose thinking about the couch and the session in *a cloud state*, I'm not trying to circumscribe a simplistic metaphor. I'm looking for ways to elucidate the complexity of the analyst's clinical work, showing the vast latent weave that traverses the distinct and singular psychic regions of each human being, together with the transferential encounter. The material of the session is always the fruit of countless condensations, with all the nuances I have tried to elucidate here.

Wouldn't a "good enough" psychoanalytic intervention be a kind of *Verdichtung*? That is, a composition that gathers infinite openings? The analyst is always composing, even if unconsciously. Excuse the rather didactic and "mathematical" example that follows, but it may help us to grasp the scale of the complexity we are discussing. Let's say an analysand speaks for 3 minutes, without interruption. In those 3 minutes, they might speak around 300 words, each of which refers to different associative representational networks, opening up associative networks of different categories that refer to images, smells, sounds, other words, experiences that refer to other experiences ... in short: the associative chain that each analysand offers the analyst, in floating attention, is infinite. If a single word can lead to countless associations, imagine 300!

After these 3 minutes, the analyst can continue in silence and listen to another 300 words (and their associations) or many more, which will be added to the first ones, or they can make an intervention/composition, using only a few elements from these 300 words and their underlying associations. For, at some level, the analyst is always composing – there is always an activity of elaborating a question or an interpretation.

Another analyst would do it differently; that is, our example contains only 3 minutes, and we are already elucidating an intervention that could very well belong to a "classical analysis". I'm not even mentioning, for example, the 45–50 minutes of a session, two or three times a week, for years. In the same way, the analysand is composing, translating into words what belongs to the realm of their infinite associations – some of which may originally be olfactory, tactile, auditory, etc. Thus, even though our examples are built from words, we know that the forms of communication in analysis transcend them.

The analyst *composes* an intervention, because any intervention means synthesising/condensing, in a few words, something that has come from countless associations that he has made internally and even unconsciously. **The psychoanalytic process is an eternal play of composition and decomposition, carried out by both analyst and analysand.** And I use the term *compose* deliberately, since the word *análysis/analysis* means decomposition into parts. In chemistry, the process of breaking down a substance into its constituent parts is the exact opposite of *synthesis*. From this perspective, the analyst's intervention/ speech would be the exact opposite of listening. The psychoanalytic clinic is built on an eternal dialectic of joint decomposition and composition between analyst and analysand. A "good enough" analytical process presupposes intense work on the part of the analyst and analysand, so that a good job of decomposition and composition can take place. **We're talking about an eternal work of *re-formation*.**

Thinking about the session and the psychoanalytic *couch/diwan* as a *cloud state* helps us to listen to the continuous movement of decomposition and composition that permeates technique. All clinical situations, regardless of the pathological factors involved, set in motion inner processes of deconstruction and construction within a third space. In other words, psychoanalytic work takes place in a third space, *a cloud state*, in which the clouds of analysand and analyst "touch" each other. The compositions/condensations of each member of the pair touch each other and activate their *creational functions*. An inner part of the analysand and an inner part of the analyst are part of a great density in constant movement, in which they unite (synthesise/condense) and separate (decompose), transferentially, all the time, every second.[7]

The density and movement of the *cloud* are conducive to all kinds of psychic mechanisms. A cloud grows, diminishes, dissipates, unleashes the fury of tornadoes, engulfs/expels another cloud, and creates every kind of *presentational* form (that which derives from latent content) to the eyes of the observer. Psychoanalysis is, above all, about working from what is *presented*, in order thereby to access what is represented.[8]

From this perspective, the analyst's "good enough" intervention is, in a sense, a *condensed* enunciation in response what they hear from the analysand's *condensation*. The analyst works with what is *presented* from the analysand's inner world and inner regions through the forms (*cloud*) and dense nebulosity of the shared third space. The optimal point for the analyst's intervention would be to offer a *condensed* content (an interpretation, for example), at the same time that this content is also *condensed* into a "good enough form", in order to converse with what the analysand has presented in their *cloud state* and, if successful, to reach and work within the analysand's Unconscious System (if we think in Freudian terms, to make it easier for the reader to understand). Therefore, the analyst's intervention must bring together both content and form.

Notes

1 Bachelard, 1990.
2 Campos, (1992) 2015, pp. 147–148.
3 Pound, 2013, p. 92.
4 Valéry, (1937/1938) 2018, p. 13.
5 Jovelina Maria Ramos de Souza presents the concept of *poíesis* in a text that details various uses for it since its origins: "An expression that originates from the verb *poiéo* (to make, execute, confect), *poíesis* is translated as manufacture, confection, preparation, production" (Souza, 2007, p. 96).
6 Shelley, (1840 [1815]) 2008, p. 77.
7 One of the many aims of this chapter is to argue how deeply each analyst's internal processes (and their theoretical presuppositions) reverberate in their interventions. Perhaps it's too early to say since the later chapters are crucial for a better understanding of the proposal, but I'm introducing the idea of a *cloud state* shared in session, which could be seen as a "meeting point" between the analysand's *cloud state* and the analyst's *cloud state*. In the case of the analyst, their technical choices and interventions (even their silence) are invariably derived from their psychic contact (their *reverie*, their countertransference, their internal relationship with themselves, their internal relationship with all their psychoanalytic studies and experiences, etc.) with the analysand's cloud state, but also from the potential capacity for their own internal *creational* movement (which involves activating their *psychic regions*). Their interventions are "drawn" from their internalities through contact with the analysand, if we may put it simply, based on what has been discussed so far (since important issues about how this would take place have not yet been contextualised). Part II, Chapter 21, "Symbolic vesture and clinical presentations in the *cloud state*", will offer a deeper exploration of this idea, adding important concepts to this understanding, but it is in Part II, Chapter 22, "The *couch/diwan* and the cloud metaphor in the clinic", that this proposal is developed in more detail.
8 The theoretical distinctions between what pertains to the order of "presentation" and what pertains to the order of "representation" will be clarified further ahead.

Chapter 21

Symbolic vesture and its clinical presentations in the *cloud state*

21.1 A brief prelude

We started with the etymology of *couch/diwan*, then followed and extended Goethe's cloud play proposal, created possibilities for thinking about a *cloud state* arising from *psychic regions*, and went on to examine various concepts, including condensation, also explaining how rethinking it influences the way we intervene in the clinic. Now we must delve into the concepts of *Verkleidung*, *Darstellung* and *symbolic vesture*, in order to then articulate all these proposals with what has been constructed around the metaphor of the cloud. These concepts will lead us to think of transference and its virtuality under the prism of a theatrical *presentation*, with its costumes (or their absence), and to connect such ideas in a way that adds to the proposal of the *divan/diwan* and of the session as a *cloud state*.

At first, it will not be possible to directly connect what will be presented below with what has been explained so far, although some of the concepts that will be discussed here have already been mentioned previously – and the attentive reader will certainly perceive the connections. However, when we reach the section "Psychic weaving – a path for thinking transference roles", there will be a greater integration between the concepts presented here and the metaphor of the cloud.

21.2 Essential reflections on *Verkleidung* (disguise/vesture) and *Darstellung* (presentation)

In Freudian theory, we see that the presentation of a psychic content always happens from a *Verkleidung*, a term that is usually translated into Portuguese as *disguise*, but which is broader and richer than that. Translating *Verkleidung* as disguise is very useful for thinking about its manifestation from the point of view of censorship, since unwanted psychic contents need a "disguise" to present themselves, but other translations of *Verkleidung* could be made, emphasising other facets of psychoanalytic practice.

DOI: 10.4324/9781003681212-24

Verkleidung also means coating. In this sense, it's something that covers an interior, protects an interior. *Kleidung* means vesture, and so *Verkleidung* is more than a disguise; it is also a fantasy, in the sense of fantasising. This brings us to an interesting point: we're talking about characters. Playing a role on stage. This is what representational content does in order to appear: it masks its original meaning. Therefore, what is presented is not what one actually is.

A dream is a scene in which the characters we see are not really what they represent. There is a performance, in the most literal and theatrical sense. It is the term *Darstellung* (*presentation*) that Freud uses to describe what is presented to us in our dreams; and yet *Darsteller* means actor. Therefore, dreams and symptoms are figurations, in the sense of performing a role, which conceal the representational content. At this point, what Freud is telling us is that the unconscious creates a play and plays tricks on us. It creates scenes and characters that, if taken literally, deceive us. At a conscious level, we only have access to this manifest content through this "play" or "masquerade". The latent content/representation itself is hidden beyond *vestures*. Freudian theory is based on scenes and tragedy, with dreams and symptoms being its main "theatres".

It is crucial to emphasise Laurence Kahn's[1] criticism of the neologisms *figurabilité/figurability/figurabilidade*, taken from a possible translation of *Darstellbarkeit* (presentability, representability), because, on a theoretical level, the term figurability is used to think about the construction of a representation via an image; above all the mental images that occur within the analyst, to be offered as support for the psychic complexification that would lead to representational paths within the analysand. At least this is how César and Sara Botella work. When I refer to the *cloud state*, I'm not necessarily referring to the concreteness of the imagetic formation, but to the whole paradoxical range of listening angles, even though the image may be an auxiliary path.

By no means is it my intention to diminish the importance of such imagetic resources in the clinic. In fact, I believe it has great importance and is complementary in any analysis, as the authors argue. However, I also believe that it is important to demarcate what *Darstellung* is and how Freud uses the term: in the sense of *taking the place of a repressed representation*. Therefore, it wouldn't be appropriate to use the term figurability, but it would be interesting to think of *figuration*, as it refers to the figurative sense and to costuming. Such a conception would preserve the original meaning of the term – differently from translating *Darstellbarkeit* as *figurability*, which is already a neologism and which would lead to different interpretations.

To figure, to impersonate, to act in a role. It is in this sense that we often see *Darstellung* also translated as representation.[2] After all, the term representation would also fit. In this sense, even though the meanings of each term may lend themselves to diverse uses, it becomes useful to reserve each term for specific situations, rather than making them analogous and undifferentiated. The difference is that we're not talking about a mental representation and/or unconscious content; we're talking about playing a role, just like an actor. From the *Spiel* and its ramifications, Freud emphasises a direct correlation between play and theatrical performance. Translator Paulo César de Souza makes a note in his translation of Freud's text *Psychopathic Characters in the Theatre*,[3] to clarify: "The word *Spiel*, which corresponds to the English word *play* …".[4] Let's see what Freud says in *The Poet and Fantasy*:

> The poet does something similar to the child who plays; he creates a fantasy world that he takes seriously, in other words, a world formed by great affective mobilisation, insofar as it is rigidly distinguished from reality. And language maintains this affinity between childish play and poetic creation, insofar as the poet's discipline, which requires the borrowing of concrete objects that can be represented, is characterised as play [*Spiele*]: comedy [*Lustspiel*], tragedy [*Trauerspiel*] and the people who represent them, as actors [*Schauspieler*].[5]

Let's read the term "representation" as "presentation",[6] due to the original word used, as explained in the note. As for the *Spiel*, translator Ernani Chaves adds:

> *Spiel*, *spielen*, play, refer to the art of acting in the theatre. So *Lustspiel* is "comedy", i.e. "a play that gives pleasure, provokes laughter, is *lustig*"; *Trauerspiel* is tragedy, i.e. "a play with something that saddens, infuriates" and *Schauspieler/in* is the "actor", the "actress", the one who "plays, plays with their appearance", according to the character.[7]

It is at this nodal point that we link children's play, poetic-making and theatre as indispensable foundations for thinking about any phenomenon or clinical practice in psychoanalysis. From the perspective of the symptom, no example is clearer than the classic hysterical symptom: conversion, a symptom that "pretends" to be organic but has a sexual aetiology. Where play is impossible, the symptom plays its trick.

Laurence Kahn points out that both dreams and symptoms are *Darstellung*. "*Darstellung* is related to the appearance under which something presents itself to perceptual consciousness."[8] **In 1897, Freud had already noted that "the mechanism of poetic creation is the same as that of hysterical fantasies",[9] and these concepts, which I have sought to weave together from the beginning, invite us to consider that my proposal to approach psychoanalytic clinic and the couch under a poetic prism is a way of continuing to develop the Freudian project.**

From the perspective of the transference, we can thus think that the analysand summons the analyst into this role-playing. Just as what is presented in the dream is not the latent content, but only the manifest content that covers it up – and the characters that make it up are basically disguises, re-vested *in symbolic vesture*. The analysand's transference to the analyst *re-vests* him in this *vesture*, just as happens in the formation of commitment that operates in dreams. Therefore, what the analysand "perceives" in the analyst is never the analyst himself; it is only the symbolic vesture with which the analysand has clothed the analyst.

In the conception being developed – from the metaphor of the cloud – the analyst's abstinent position places him as an amorphous material, an amorphous cloud, yet malleable, to be re-vested for the play of transferential staging to which the analysand summons him. The analyst is seen according to what the analysand's cloud state – which permeates the cloud state shared in the session – has re-vested him with and will re-vest him with incessantly, in all the ways necessary for his process of analysis.

21.3 The *symbolic vesture*: a conceptualisation

It is now essential to deepen the important concept of *symbolic vesture*, which was mentioned earlier without sufficient space for proper elucidation.

When we were translating[10] Karl Abraham's book *Dream and Myth: A Study in the Psychology of Peoples*[11] (1909) and discussing the various possibilities of translation, we realised that Abraham emphasised the allegorical character, but above all the notions of vestures and re-vesting inherent in the word *Verkleidung*. His theorising is based on gradations of covering in contrast to what would be naked stories, naked words. I'll give you two examples in a footnote, among other possible ones.[12]

More than that, Abraham uses the compound term *symbolische Verkleidung*, which we prefer to translate as *symbolic vesture* – and I intend to explain why. His entire theoretical construction of myths, based mainly on the theory of sexuality and the interpretation of dreams, carries the idea of *symbolic vesture*. For our purposes here, Abraham essentially talked about more-or-less "naked" myths.

The closer the manifest content of the myth – that is, the way it is told – approached the latent and sexual content, the more "naked" this myth would be. The more *symbolic vesture* (*symbolische Verkleidung*) this myth had, the more distant it would be from accessing the unconscious representation. Consequently, the closer the mythological narrative was to the unconscious representation, with fewer "disguises," the more Abraham would point to its nakedness and rawness.

The difficulty in deconstructing a myth into its unconscious character seems to be proportional to the amount of *symbolic vesture*. Therefore, the greater the difficulty in breaking down the myth into its unconscious and sexual character, the more "cloaked" in *symbolic vesture* the myth would be. The form of this *vesture* would depend on all the psychic mechanisms that help to make it, including displacement and condensation.

Abraham's theoretical proposal is to demonstrate the sexual character of myths. When he refers to the nakedness and rawness of a myth, he always refers to its proximity to sexual and incestuous content, echoing Freud's propositions. Although it is fundamentally important to think of nudity from the point of view of sexuality, I believe we can also borrow the term *symbolic vesture* for use in another context.

I justify this because, as translators, if we were to follow the tradition of translating *Verkleidung* into Portuguese, it would be usual to translate Abraham's compound term as "symbolic disguise". In our psychoanalytic tradition, the primacy of the word disguise for *Verkleidung* is indisputable; nevertheless we have presented an alternative translation that is also consistent with its meaning. *Kleidung* strictly means vesture, and Abraham works theoretically in contrast to nakedness and rawness. Therefore, I believe that, within this context, *symbolic vesture* would make it even easier for the Portuguese-speaking reader to understand the plurality of meanings offered by Abraham when using the term (taking into account what I explained earlier about the richness of the term *Verkleidung* transcending the notion of disguise).

Every translation is subject to interpretation and choice: depending on the expression being translated, one meaning or another may be favoured. Therefore, translating the word *Verkleidung* as *vesture*, outside of the context used by Abraham, contains a certain boldness. I believe our reading of the context diminished this boldness in translation, since it would move towards a better understanding of Abraham's proposal as a whole. Nevertheless, we cannot deny that we relied on some authoriality in creating the term *symbolic vesture* (in Portuguese, *roupagem simbólica*).

It is at this point, where there is a dose of authoriality in composing the expression in Portuguese, that I feel compelled to take another bold step: to appropriate this terminology from a re-actualised perspective. It seems interesting to me to use the term *symbolic vesture* also in the context of non-neurotic sufferings, if we carry out the idea of contrasting what would belong to the order of nakedness, of rawness, with what would be of an order of representational layers.

In non-predominantly neurotic cases, instead of thinking of nakedness from the point of view of sexuality – naturally prevailing in theorisations of 1909 – we would take "nakedness" and "rawness" as what would be of the order of the traumatic, the mortifying, the torturous, the disorganizing, what is left bare.[13] In such circumstances, the analyst's work would be to help the analysand weave and/or put on *symbolic vesture* in order to get out of the cruel cold of pain. To make pain re-vest itself in costumes[14] and act in a play (in the clinical realm, transferentially), and not in the analysand's life outside the consulting room. To transform this pain through the transferential use of these symbolic vestures.

The *symbolic vesture* is an aid to clinical listening as, from it, the characters and plays that need to be staged are dramatised in session. This proposal contextualises and actualises what Freud wrote about working *per via di porre* and *per via di levare*.[15] The transferential field is a continuous "taking off, putting on, and changing vesture/figurine". Sometimes the work of analysis is weaving and wrapping; it's stripping off the immense layers of costume that hide what's behind.

More than 100 years after Abraham's text, when we psychoanalysts use the adjectives "naked" and "raw", we are often no longer referring primarily to sexuality, as Abraham did. We are talking about destructive acts (storms, hurricanes, in our metaphor *of* the *cloud state*). If we think of the width of the *couch/ diwan* from its function as customs house and as meeting room, we are thinking of it as the third space where the *clouds* of analyst and analysand meet. In this case, one of the analyst's missions is to attempt to contain the analysand's stormy and destructive cloud, offering in return a clearer cloud that is more willing to filter out disruptive excess. The analyst will receive and welcome the other person's destructiveness so that, together, they can transform it into something creative. In this way, psychoanalytic work, gradually realised from a shared *cloud state*, would indirectly develop the analysand's most damaged *psyche regions* in a healthy way.

21.4 Psychic weaving – a path for thinking transference roles

Having explained the concepts of *presentation* and *symbolic vesture*, let's return to the ludic trail and the importance of *play* (*Spiel*) that I've been emphasising. We can use the malleability of the cloud figure in various ways, including the cloud as cotton, a raw material for weaving clothes. Yes, let's play with the playfulness of this idea, without repressing it beforehand. Mark Strand[16] might say: "Clouds in wardrobes become clothes" and "At sunset, the clouds put on their dresses and step out into the night".

Weaving happens through interlaced threads. Let us think that this interlacing, this entanglement, is made of threads. Let us take the cotton cloud as an allegory that encompasses this aspect of psychic weaving, which is fundamental to our reflection. In *The Interpretation of Dreams* (1900),[17] in the chapter dedicated to the mechanism of condensation, Freud cites *Faust*, by Goethe,[18] to present the movements of the Unconscious as a weaving machine, which condenses threads and creates connections.

> *Each pedal stroke moves a thousand threads,*
> *the shuttles fly back and forth,*
> *the threads flow unseen,*
> *one strike creates a thousand bonds.*[19]

In this specific poetic image, which Freud used precisely to explain the psychic mechanism of condensation, we might emphasize the loom[20] and the connections allied to the aforementioned act of "flying/floating", which are closely connected to what was previously articulated about the suspension of clouds, as well as what was said about *Verdichtung* (condensation) and the *Dichter* (poet). It's also important to point out that *Faust* is a play, written as a long dramatic poem, and that, in the passage selected, both Goethe and Freud tell us about movements, cloud play, invisible threads that build plots and figurations. From the perspective I want to elucidate, the *cloud* (shared in session) lends itself to being both the stage/theatre and the fabric/cotton present in the *diwan*. It seems to me that elevating the analytical session into a *cloud state*, in the sense of floating, emphasises the malleability of internal movement and the roles dramatised in the transference.

Translator Luiz Hanns draws attention to how Freudian conceptualisation takes place and Freud's use of words when creating his basic terminology. Hanns[21] points out that all Freud's theoretical concepts have an intricate semantic-theoretical network. Each concept naturally leads to another, and many of the translations we are used to in Portuguese cause the original semantic-conceptual relationship to be lost.

Therefore, the following theoretical elucidations revolve around theatre, since this is the semantic thread upon which Freud relies from the outset, even though it is possible to weave equivalent thoughts from cinema.

Unlike cinema, however, theatre offers us a time of amorphous waiting when the scene changes. The lights go out, smoke billows and dazzles the spectator, like a cloud when one form has vanished and another has yet to emerge. As happens in the transferential play, when the analyst is just "amorphous" (a non-role in the transferential play) waiting for the new psychic movements of the session to clothe him in some *symbolic vesture*, thus enabling him to take part in the "play" necessary for that particular analysis. In other words, the transferential role that the analyst occupies in the analysis of an analysand is not static. They can, for example, occupy one transferential role at a given moment in a session, and then occupy another. There is always movement. Like a wind (drive?) that gives the cloud form (offering it a *symbolic vesture*) but then removes it, dissipates it, leaving the analyst amorphous within the transferential field, until a new *symbolic vesture* is once again offered.

From this perspective, the *shared cloud state* (as a third space of exchange and contact between the analysand's cloud and the analyst's cloud)[22] that permeates the atmosphere of the session, coming from the analysand's *psychic regions*, and which summons the analyst's *psychic regions* to the analytic work, "offers" transferential roles that *are presented* from a scene that is established in the session (similar to what Freud would call transference neurosis), in favour of the development of the psychoanalytic work. In other words, what I call the *cloud state* is nothing more than a potential amorphous state, or rather, a substance in constant movement, which doesn't have a univocal form. As the psychoanalytic process develops, *symbolic vestures* are *presented* and woven. Later, they dissipate, are woven again, and so on. From this perspective, the *couch/diwan* and the *cloud state* that is intrinsic to it function as a stage for the transferential play.

It's important to emphasise that I don't see this proposition as simply starting from an internal theatre, which takes place within each person. This proposal differs from Joyce McDougall's proposal of a "stage",[23] since when she refers to the terms "theatre" and "stage", she is always referring to the individual, and not to the psychoanalytic atmosphere as a whole. McDougall wants to think of the internal world and the body as a stage and theatre of oneself. **Our proposal, however, adopts an intersubjective perspective: the transferential play is conceived as a theatrical (and thus virtual) *Spiel* (play), in which the stage is the couch–diwan–cloud – that is, the consulting room as a whole, along with its virtual atmosphere.** In this case, the analyst is transferentially *re-vested* in a *symbolic vesture* and is part of the scene necessary for the analytical process in question. In the paradox of this thought, the *cloud-couch/diwan* both weaves and is the stage – whether of representations or of himself. The *couch/diwan*, the "important meeting" room of the analysis as a whole, is a simulacrum of a stage (as we mentioned earlier), allowing the clouds of each member of the analytical pair to move in this third space of contact, which is the psychoanalytic session itself.

If Freud explains to us that "Condensation, together with the transformation of thoughts into situations ('dramatisation') is the most important and peculiar characteristic of dream work",[24] and this occurs within everyone, let's transpose Freud's reflection on internal functioning to what would be analogous to the intersubjective context of the session, since everything that Freud points out would also take place on the "stage" of the session, within the *shared cloud state*.

Notes

1 Khan, 2016.
2 This is the case in the *Complete Works of Freud* published by Imago (derived from the English translation by James Strachey) and in the direct translations from the German by Paulo César de Souza. See Freud, 1974; Freud, 2010; Freud, 1953–1974.
3 Freud, (1942 [1905/1906]) 2019a, p. 362.
4 Freud, (1942 [1905/1906]) 2019a, p. 363. In Portuguese, there is no single word that covers the full semantic range of *Spiel* or *play*. In the Brazilian edition, this point was explained in more detail, but here a shorter version will suffice.
5 Freud, (1908a [1907]) 2015a, p. 54.
6 As we can see from the German original and the words in bold (*Darstellung* and *darstellt*), although the translation uses "representation" – and, in fact, this term does exist in theatre and refers to the actor's work – Freud's original sentence points more precisely to what concerns "presentation", not an unconscious representation. It refers to the way in which one content is presented through another. From the point of view of Freudian metapsychology, we could say that the "presentation" derives from unconscious representations, but it is not analogous to them; it is simply the form in which they are presented, whether in a dream, a symptom, an artistic work or a play. This distinction is important so that the reader does not confuse their understanding of metapsychology. At times, when the reader encounters the

word "representation" in the Portuguese versions, it is used in the sense of "unconscious representation"; at other times it is used in the sense of the "presentation" we are discussing here.

Here is the original: "Und die Sprache hat diese Verwandtschaft von Kinderspiel und poetischem Schaffen festgehalten, indem sie solche Veranstaltungen des Dichters, welche der Anlehnung an greibare Objekte bedürfen, welche der **Darstellung** fähig sind, als Spiele: Lustspiel, Trauerspiel, und die Person, welche sie **darstellt**, als Schauspieler bezeichnet."

7 Freud, (1908b [1907]) 2015a, p. 65.
8 Kahn, 2016, p. 179.
9 Freud, 2015, p. 43.
10 This translation was carried out by Eduardo Spieler, Sander Machado da Silva and myself.
11 Abraham, (1909) 2020.
12 Here are two (non-consecutive) paragraphs from Abraham, 2020, both on page 23:

> The legends [Abraham does not differentiate between legends, myths and tragedies in his work] of Oedipus, Uranus and their derivatives are interrelated not only in their content, but also in their external form. In both there is an almost total lack of symbolic vesture. We experience the whole story through bare words. It's important to note that this is also true of the typical dream that we'll use to explain these myths. They contain – as Freud observes – the symbolic vesture in a surprising formation.
>
> Censorship does not allow our most secret desires to express themselves in dreams in a naked, raw and undisguised way (*unverhüllten*). On the contrary, it forces desires to obscure their true tendency by *distorting* them in the dream. The diversion of censorship is realised through extensive *dream work*. We'll consider its manifestations in more detail later. For now, let's just deal with the dream's form of distortion – the symbolic vesture of desire.

13 Or what would be falsely cloaked, like the Winnicottian *false self*, for example.
14 It would be interesting to think about the proposal to "clothe" suffering naked and raw, relating it to Didier Anzieu's comments (see Part I, Chapter 4, "Didier Anzieu's skin couch") about analysands who seek to create more "layers of skin", using blankets in session, or even over-warming themselves – a resource employed by many psychotics to maintain a degree of psychic integration.
15 The contexts need to be differentiated here. Freud uses the terms to describe what would be the order of suggestion (*per via de porre*) and what would be classical analysis, decomposition (*per via de levare*). I take the idea of *per via de porre* from the point of view of representational construction, not from the point of view of suggestion [Freud, (1905 [1904]) 1989].
16 Strand, 2016. *Another poetic vision of the thoughts that follow could be*: "If you prefer, I'll just be mad meat / and, like the sky, I'll change my tune if you prefer, / I'll be impeccably delicate, / I won't be a man, but a cloud of trousers!" – Vladimir Mayakovski (1995).
17 Freud, (1900) 2019.
18 Goethe, 2012.
19 Freud, (1900) 2019, p. 324.
20 In *The Interpretation of Dreams*, Freud also refers to the fabric of the dream [Freud, (1900) 2019, p. 615].
21 Hanns, 2016, pp. 176–182.
22 Refer back to Part II, Chapter 19, "The psychic regions and the cloud state", to understand how this "cloud formation" in the psyche takes place.
23 McDougall, (1982) 1989; (1989) 1996.
24 Freud, (1901) 1996c, pp. 672–673.

Chapter 22

The couch/*diwan* and the cloud metaphor in the clinic

22.1 Returning to the proposal of *psychic regions* to think about the clinic

I'll begin this chapter by reiterating that the metaphor *of psychic regions* is not intended to create a map of how the Unconscious works, nor is it intended to inaugurate a new metapsychology. Rather, it serves as an auxiliary theoretical-clinical construct to support listening in analysis, and it remains attentive to the multiplicity of understandings within the various ways of conceiving the analytic process.

I'm not postulating here exactly what these imagined and hypothetical *psychic regions* would be like, but perhaps it's possible to consider different versions of them, as some authors have endeavoured to do in similar proposals, as mentioned in Chapter 19, "The psychic regions and the cloud state". We could think of them in terms of psychopathological zones, but we could also think of them terms of what Bollas discusses, in terms of psychoanalytic theories being internal objects for the analyst, which he can use as auxiliary tools for listening. Transposed to the proposal of *psychic regions*, this perspective would imply that each psychoanalytic theory could be thought of as a kind of internal country – but not only within the analyst. In this view, the internal world of the analysand would itself be inhabited by all these "theoretical countries", each with its singular mode of psychic mapping and its own language.[1]

It would also be possible to consider these regions based on forms of psychic functioning similar to the erogenous zones proposed by Freud. Thus, we could envisage an internal region of an oral-anal nature, which would operate on the basis of mechanisms such as incorporation, expulsion, introjection, projection and projective identification. Another region would operate on the basis of compromise formations and would produce returns of the repressed; there would also be a third, empty, desert region.

That said, no postulation could ever suffice to encompass the psychic depths in their entirety, for, in the end, not even Freud succeeded in constructing a theory without considerable gaps. Let's assume our incompleteness in this

DOI: 10.4324/9781003681212-25

regard. The fact remains that, even if we cannot (and do not intend to) specify these *psychic regions* directly, the idea that from them arises the 'deep water' giving rise to the *cloud state* – presenting itself in the session – seems to me a fruitful way of thinking the multiplicity of listening and intervening in the clinic.

If we are to conceive the analysand's psyche in terms of diverse *psychic regions*, which present themselves in session through the *cloud state* and the *symbolic vesture* that compose it, then our task differs from listening through a specific psychopathological structure or a single theoretical vertex. After all, each theoretical vertex presents a different kind of map of how the psyche might function.

Our listening thus aims, above all, to identify which psychic mechanism is operating at any given moment of the analysis. Certainly, some mechanisms will manifest themselves more than others in each process of analysis. However, it wouldn't be helpful to think that each and every communication from the analysand manifests itself through the same route. We are never free from receiving communications that come from psychotic or arid, empty regions, even if neurotic regions predominate in an analysand. The reverse would also be true – that is to say, all psychic regions would be part of an "immense Unconscious".[2]

22.2 Psychic defence mechanisms and predominantly neurotic *internal regions*

Although I have explained the *symbolic vesture* from a predominantly neurotic perspective, considering the model of the dream, we must admit that a delirium, for example, is also presented in a *symbolic vesture* to cover something up. The *symbolic vesture* would be the product *presented*, regardless of the defence mechanisms that led to its production. And we could think of it as the product of the "return" of all kinds of structuring cleavages,[3] such as repression (*Verdrängung*), rejection (*Verwerfung*) and denial (*Verleugnung*):[4] defence mechanisms that Freud links to neuroses, psychoses and perversions, respectively, although his thinking is not as simplistic as it is summarised here.

What matters here is to highlight the range of "structuring" mechanisms that are juxtaposed, especially if we add those described by Freud to the thoughts and conceptualisations of the other authors who were presented earlier. Still thinking from Freud's point of view, let's remember that he presents the "man of the wolves"[5] as an obsessive neurosis, but he also tells us that, at some level, a rejection (*Verwerfung*) of castration was at work. This case, which was later attended to by Ruth Mack Brunswick, was diagnosed by her as hypochondria and paranoia (a pathology to which Freud related Schreber's psychosis),[6] and is a case that has been the subject of discussion about its diagnosis to this day, including positions that understand it as borderline. When dealing with Mrs P,[7] Freud also speaks of "hallucinatory paranoia"[8] and "depression" filled with delusions and hallucinations, coexisting concomitantly with a neurotic obsessional-neurotic symptomatology, as well as to a "repression through projection"[9] operating alongside "normal" repressions – if indeed one may call them that.

If we don't focus on fitting the case into a psychodiagnostic frame, we stand a better chance of apprehending the vast internal world at stake. I believe we are dealing with psychic regions (internal parts with diverse modes of functioning) that coexist in the internal world, existing in juxtaposition as they interrelate and *present* themselves. It is undeniable that the "man of the wolves" had neurotic-obsessive symptoms, as Freud thought, but perhaps not just because he inhabited a more complex universe than a simplifying psychopathological nosography.

How, then, are we to understand the hallucinations and hysterical delusions described by Freud? There are mentions of these psychic occurrences, for example, in the cases of Mrs Emy Von N., Anna O. and Dora, as well as in Freud's more general descriptions of hysterical phenomena.[10] How should we think of them? Freud is certainly not talking about psychotic structures; he presents us with delusions and hallucinations as natural symptoms of hysteria, commenting on these delusions as products of internal conflicts and compromise formations. We could ask ourselves, based on contemporary clinical practice, how often we come across delusions and hallucinations (and how we should view them), but that's not the point. We have to think that at that time Freud was dealing primarily with hysteria, and he had not yet postulated the concept of narcissism. He was dealing with unconscious incestuous desire of the girl/woman's infantile sexuality for her father.

Christopher Bollas,[11] in his book *Hysteria*,[12] seeks to integrate the hysterical phenomenon through what he conceives as a constitutive primary narcissism:[13] the baby's relationship with the mother (its maternal function) and the way in which this primary narcissism relates to the "Oedipus Complex proper (Freudian)" and the desires and conflicts inherent in it. In his book, Bollas's concern is to show that, nowadays, many of the cases that were being treated by psychoanalysts as borderline cases could and should be understood within the field of hysteria. The re-reading of hysteria proposed by Bollas, which also brings narcissistic-primitive aspects into the debate, helps us to think about the idea of internal psychic regions and how their modes of functioning interrelate (and are presented from the point of view of the *cloud state* and *symbolic vestures*).

In this line of reasoning, it is important to remember that there is no type of neurosis that is not initially based on a structuring primary narcissistic foundation (and primitive forms of functioning). Freud presents us with the hallucinatory fulfilment of desire[14] as constitutive of the psyche (and the basis of the dream model), hallucination being naturally constitutive and a type of operating mode of the psyche present in every human being. In a primitive moment, obviously, hallucination and delirium are equivalent, since the baby hallucinates the breast, "believing" (of the order of delirium) in its presence. Furthermore, in *The Interpretation of Dreams*, Freud relates psychoses to the dream state,[15] helping us to understand that phenomena that we could call psychotic and psychotic defence mechanisms are the founding basis of any and all psychisms.[16]

So, if the hallucinatory fulfilment of desire (which holds within itself a *creational* potential – an active and omnipotent movement that creates something) plays an important role in the foundation of a psyche, there's no way of saying that primitive defence mechanisms aren't at work in some *internal regions* of oneself, even if they don't *present* themselves or don't manifest themselves as sources of suffering.

Not even if we were talking about someone whose functioning is predominantly neurotic, we cannot fail to consider the existence of internal areas operating through more primitive or psychotic mechanisms. This would be one of the possible explanations for the imminence of delusions and hallucinations in clinical cases that we can't call psychotic, like Freud's neurotic cases – in which hallucinations and delusions *present themselves*. In cases like these, a type of functioning (procedural, not necessarily a content)[17] of a primitive order would "combine" with the incestuous oedipal conflict (if we're talking about hysteria), *presenting* some delirium (or hallucination).

> For the hallucinations of hysteria, paranoia and the visions of normal-minded people, I can explain that they really correspond to regressions, that is to say, thoughts transformed into images, and that only thoughts closely linked to repressed memories or that have remained unconscious undergo this transformation.[18]

Delusional/hallucinatory phenomena predominate in psychotics; however, because these phenomena are constitutive of every human being, they also end up *appearing* in hysteria and obsessive neurosis (as in Freud's cases), as well as in other types of psychic suffering that we could not classify as a predominantly psychotic structure. These phenomena can become part of the session and the transferential field in a more intense or less intense way, as analysis and the use of the couch naturally lead to regression/regredience in order to evoke what needs to be worked on. The couch and the analysis session instrumentally lead to regressions,[19] although in some cases these can be more "profound" or disturbing than others. The whole psychoanalytic process involves processes of regression/regression.

Therefore, during the listening process, it is essential to listen to the psychic defence mechanism that is at work at that moment, based on the *cloud state* and the *symbolic vestures* presented. For example, again, a hysteric or an obsessive neurotic could possibly, at some point in their analysis, try to incorporate the analyst, as happens in the oral-cannibalistic phase proposed by Abraham.[20]

They could deny what they have experienced, manifest some psychotic facet or deposit traumatised internal areas into the session. I am convinced that the psychoanalytic reader has already come across situations similar to these, because they are "expected" to present themselves in an analysis process.

22.3 The couch and its relevance to clinical work beyond neurosis

I made a point of problematising the face-to-face, even in Part I, while bringing in the contributions of other authors, since in my clinical practice the couch has not been an obstacle to good analytical work, regardless of the type of psychopathological suffering of my analysands. On the contrary, it has been my ally, even in situations that border on depersonalisation and the risk of suicide. From the moment I began to reflect on the range of its functions, supported by the authors I worked with earlier, I began to recommend it as soon as the initial interviews were completed and a work contract was signed. However, this appointment does not take place without a prior dialogue, without me explaining to the analysand why I am using this instrument-object as an aid to their analysis. I will comment on this throughout this section.

Nothing would prevent me from reconsidering my current position on this, but I believe that the way in which the analyst sees the work from the couch is more important than thinking about its use or non-use *a priori*. Much of what has already been said supports this position. My work with children probably "helps" me to take the couch-object more broadly. It would be simplistic to think of its use only through the prism of a classical analysis. Supporting the use of the couch in analyses that involve non-neurotic predominances goes through several vertices that we presented earlier, especially from Ferenczi, Winnicott, Ogden and Bollas, as well as the other authors mentioned. I deeply respect colleagues who have other experiences that would lead them to disagree with my current position, but I can only speak from my clinical practice.[21]

With regard to working with analysands in whom aspects of the neurotic order dominate, I don't think I have anything new to add here (that hasn't already been discussed), except to emphasise the importance of what relates to the pleasure of playing in session (although not in the same way as a child) as a springboard to help loosen the bonds of the neuroses that bind these analysands. Since the beginning of psychoanalysis, the couch has been an aid in the treatment of neuroses, and everything that has been presented and discussed so far makes the importance of its use unquestionable. I certainly carry all the contributions of the authors mentioned above into my listening.

As for working with analysands who suffer from non-neurotic ailments, with each passing year I become more convinced of the importance of the couch. Of course, I don't treat anyone in an outburst situation, where a psychotic peak prevents any kind of communication, but the moments when psychotic or depersonalising aspects manifest themselves during analyses – including with analysands in whom there is a neurotic predominance – don't seem to me to be an obstacle to health.

However, I would reiterate that in no way do I wish to invalidate the importance of face-to-face treatments (or any other modality that does away with the couch). I couldn't possibly do so, not least because part of my psychoanalytic training took place at the São Pedro Psychiatric Hospital in Porto Alegre, one of the oldest public hospitals (formerly called hospices) in the country, where cases of extremely severe psychosis are dealt with and where the use of the couch is obviously not even considered. The purpose of this book is to discuss psychoanalytic treatments in spaces where it is possible to use the couch as a resource, such as consulting rooms.

I believe it is the analyst's task to tolerate the dive into the most destructive aspects that working on the couch can lead to. As for my colleagues who criticise the use of the couch and avoid it on the grounds that it could lead the analysand to disintegrative experiences in analysis, I believe they are right in part of their reasoning. In fact, if there is an internal need for the analysand to relive, repair, re-stitch some primitive aspect of themselves, the work on the couch will help them to "descend" to the respective *psychic regions* of more primitive functioning. Would that be undesirable? Couldn't it be part of the treatment that the analysand has a kind of primitive transference with the figure of the analyst and with the other inanimate objects in the consulting room, especially with the couch, which could be *re-vested symbolically* as the mother's body?[22]

Some analysands fall asleep in session and experience soothing feelings, in which regressions to maternal dependencies (in the sense of watching over and protecting) are clearly manifested. These are situations in which the analysand seeks the analyst's presence from the couch, a certain internal peace. They psychically merge the couch with the figure of the analyst as a protective and *holding* function. In these cases, working on the couch becomes a kind of reparation, the re-stitching of wounded "holes" in the self.

After and during the sessions in which these episodes of falling asleep occur, the analysand often brings up apparently disconnected contents and/or ways of functioning which, over time, make a certain sense within a non-sense. These are difficult situations to exemplify, not least because many of them are experienced silently, within the analysand,[23] while some are shared in the third space. They are situations beyond the reach of words.

Taking Ogden's propositions, we could say that a large part of these experiences takes place only privately, within the analysand, and part of this experience is incommunicable, unspeakable to the analyst, who participates in some of these moments only as a witness who can "understand" what is happening in session from his *reverie*.

This is not a matter of the analyst attempting to interpret something that occurs within a regressive context; it is rather a matter of respecting the moment, experiencing the transferential role that has been placed upon him or her and exercising their *container* function. Depending on the situation, the analyst, as the mother-couch-object, should at most appease the analysand and reassure them that they are in a protected environment, if necessary. Any work to re-elaborate what has been lived, re-lived, takes place *a posteriori*, in subsequent sessions and from the internal time that the analysand signals.

I'm referring here to visiting the border between being and not being. In the same way that the analyst never deals directly with the repressed content of a neurosis – but only touches on it from what is *presented* in session – neither does he reach the factuality of primitive scenes. His participation and his "understanding" depend on his *reverie*. I have my doubts about whether concrete examples would help us understand these propositions, because these regressive moments don't always occur in radical forms, but I'll try to elucidate them in some way.[24]

There have been situations in analysis in which I was desperately called "mother" after long silences and/or slumbers, and although the analysands then realised their "slip" and tried to convey to me what they were experiencing internally, these are situations that words cannot reach. It's *as if* something is only transmitted to the analyst on a sensory level, and *as if* it's only through an unspoken pathway that the analysand is able to communicate with me.

Analysands often also report feeling "embraced" by the couch, which became a problem during the pandemic (and the shift from in-person to online treatment), as the couch's function bodily continuity was broken in some cases. Although analysands reported missing the couch a lot and relating its "loss" to a feeling of missing something in themselves, other analysands, who also took the couch as an object that exercised this maternal function on a deeper level, became more confused. They depended on me to help them more actively (among other analytical functions) to understand and state that, in fact, there had been a sudden break in the texture-*holding* that the couch provided as a support for their psyche during the work of analysis.

After introspective silences, analysands can report seeing themselves outside of themselves; feeling "joined" to the couch; feeling like they are floating. They often communicate originary sensations, whether of fusion and de-fusion of themselves, or of being at ease, but also of intrusion – which means that the analyst's handling involves bringing in aspects of material reality, beyond the psychic, to ensure the analytic space as a safe place for the analysand. Experiencing situations in analysis that are analogous to not-being oneself is also a path of connecting to primary creativity (by creating one's world and oneself) – what I've been referring to as the *creational* order. In the sense of accessing a *creational* state: in a way, reviving the original sensation of creating oneself, in the work of *re-formation* that is analysis.

As for the analysand feeling invaded and reporting some sensation akin to being invaded, attacked, or "swallowed up" by the couch, I think this works in our favour. After all, if these are internal issues to be worked through, it is in fact preferable that they be directed and transferred onto the couch-object – an inanimate third object (much like a toy in child analysis) – rather than onto the analyst.[25] In a face-to-face consultation, invasiveness would be transferentially linked massively to the person of the analyst.

Of course, on the couch, the analysand will also transfer to the analyst, but mediated by a thirdness that would, to say the least, be disrupted if the treatment took place face-to-face. On the couch, certainly, some analysands may imagine that the analyst is mocking their feelings and imagine, more neurotically (or even psychotically), that the analyst would harm them, expel them, destroy them, or submit them to some form of abuse – any situation belonging to the order of abuse and the absence of alterity. These are issues intrinsically linked to their narcissistic constitution, and they really need to be worked on.

When I recommend the couch, I always warn the analysand beforehand that, at some point in the process of analysis, they may have unsettling or disturbing feelings towards me (the analyst). However, I make it clear that this is entirely natural, since they will be transferring their whole life into the space of the session. I indicate that, should such a strange or unpleasant feeling occur, they should communicate it to me, and together we will attempt to understand what is taking place. After all, my primary intention as their analyst is to help them work through internally whatever their psyche shows to be necessary – and never the opposite. This is an anchoring warning that helps (and, in my practice, rarely fails[26]) whenever a negative transference, especially a more massive one, takes hold of the sessions. It is a warning-sign, a guardian warning, reminding the analysand that analysis may arouse "mad" or unpleasant feelings – and that it is perfectly acceptable for them to occur, since what matters is that we think them through together afterwards, in order to work them through.

It's a way of announcing the virtuality of what is experienced in session – showing, from the outset, that analysis takes place in a territory of "*as if*", and not of a concrete relationship. At the same time, it is something that circumscribes the analytical space as a place where psychisms dialogue; a space where dissatisfaction, destructiveness and some possible violent bodily acts are contained, or "content" themselves with being expressed in the most symbolic way possible, without the analyst suffering any physical aggression (if we think of extreme cases) or the analysand simply interrupting treatment because of an uncommunicated transferential annoyance.

Primitive uses of the couch-object can be long, but they are often brief. It can be conducive to the emergence of a certain "momentary madness", which will be better understood below. There are also analysands who, for much of their analysis – or for a given period – make use of blankets, envelopes that wrap their whole body. I understand some of these situations as analogous to Winnicott's couch-womb, since the use of the couch can be seen as a kind of protection for self-creation, protection for being, protection against invasion – even though I have never witnessed a regression as profound as those Margaret

Little describes in her analysis with Winnicott. Often, the use of the blanket serves (in the sense of being used, as an object) to protect a fragile psychic skin from trauma, from the fragility of the border between the *self* and the external world that attacks it. The blanket "embodies" this psychic skin-function.[27] In this sense, the couch is also a protection against the analyst's gaze, which would invade the analysand's psyche in a face-to-face treatment. However, blankets are also often used for "transitional" purposes, analogous to reptiles that shed their skin. In reality, human beings also shed their skin, since our cells die and are renewed at every moment.[28]

There is always a renewal and a *re-formation* of our bodies too. In such cases, blankets are offered in order to protect the "shedding" and the "composition" of a new (psychic) skin, and they serve the process of *re-formation*, as we have been articulating.

As for the use of a blanket as an auxiliary element in the analytical process on the couch, it is true that for a long time I didn't make this resource available. This demand, however, gradually arose from the words of some analysands, who began to express the wish to cover themselves during sessions. This led me to offer the possibility of their bringing their own blankets, to be kept in the consulting room cabinet, just as we store boxes and toys for children, to be used by them during their sessions.[29] Such an understanding later led me to make a blanket visibly available in the room for those who felt compelled to use it.

The criticism that using the couch can arouse persecutory and paranoid thoughts – and therefore shouldn't be recommended – sounds a bit exaggerated to me. This type of symptomatology appears in face-to-face treatments too. In fact, in a face-to-face modality, the analysand would have more support to "negatively" support their fantasies or persecutory and paranoid delusions. If the analyst appears tired or sleepy (whether this is true or not), the analysand will use this "surface" to project the idea that the analyst is not interested in them. If the analysand eventually looks at the clock, it could feel as if the analyst is counting down the hours to get rid of the "boring" analysand ... In this way, the analyst would have to work with a false "poker face", which would be terrible, or their spontaneous "humanity" could be interpreted through a paranoid lens, if such a mode of suffering were prominent in the analysand.

As in the expression "damned if you do, damned if you don't", there is no way of avoiding persecutory fantasies. They need to be confronted and, from this point of view, the couch, cutting off the gaze and the need to trust (even if distrust remains), means that these fantasies present themselves in a way that can be contained and worked through in session. Certainly, the analysand may think any absurdity about the analyst, or about what the analyst might be doing and/or thinking while the analysand is deprived of seeing them; yet the analysand will be more impelled to communicate their paranoia while lying on the couch than to "look for something" in the analyst's body that could "substantiate" it, thus living it silently without directly communicating it. Furthermore, when any kind of feeling or thought intensifies, the analysand lying on the couch can always turn their head and find the figure of the analyst, which happens when there is an internal need to reassure them of the analyst's "good" presence in session.

A 45-year-old analysand,[30] dominated by paranoid psychic regions and permeated by projective mechanisms, but also presenting other very arid psychic regions,[31] although maintaining a functional (and neurotic) side of herself, was affected by eating disorders and manifested moments of disconnection of an autistic nature (her only son had severe autism). She used to turn round to look at me many times during the session. This was her first treatment in any kind of psychotherapy. Until then, she had been undergoing psychiatric treatment for over 20 years, using only medication for depression and anxiety. Her analysis sessions were tense and her laughs were nervous, disconnected from the content – seeming scarcely genuine, as though they were a kind of attempt at existing, albeit in a schizoid mode, rather than an authentic expression of humour.

She displayed a disturbed sense of humour. On the couch, she often turned round, always looking frightened, and persecuted herself with her own words. However, all this symptomatology subsided as the treatment progressed. She started to bring a bottle of water to drink during the session (which other analysands also do, for multiple reasons, including to "lubricate" their speech)[32] and started to wear more colourful clothes, since for a long time she had only worn black and grey,[33] making a visual change from what appeared to be "death" to something she herself acknowledged and upon which she eventually reflected.

Her erotic transference demarcated her desire, but her fantasy often placed me less as a straight man (in her fantasies, I was often seen as homosexual) and more as a nurturing mother. I was a "straight man" (in the transferential role) only in her persecutory fantasies, where she transferentially regarded me as a tyrannical misogynist. In these fantasies, I would occupy the role of the bad man, who exploits her and serves her only to steal her money. Since her perception was purely transferential and not connected to anything concrete that took place in the sessions, after a certain period her transference would once again turn me into a "homosexual man" – "excessively sensitive", in her words.

Working with her was exhausting. I felt sucked dry of my psychic energies, as if she were nourishing herself on me. It took a lot of patience to receive her attacks and defuse her persecution with due benevolence and a naturally calm tone of voice, which always came out spontaneously in interventions with her. It was *as if* my psyche chewed up the terrifying world she projected and gave it back with tenderness and warmth. There was a time when she slept through most of the sessions and snored deeply (on one of these occasions, when she woke up, she told me: "*Sorry, Mum. I was so tired, I ended up blacking out*").

The subject of her sessions was often oral, involving her body weight, her binge eating, her metabolic problems and her lactose allergy. It also involved historical and cultural issues of colonisation, abuse of power and the way indigenous people were exploited in Brazil; as well as her autistic son and her relationship with her husband (who suffered from morbid obesity and severe paranoia, which made him avoid going out), as well as other aspects of her personal history. Although I was psychically exhausted by attending to her, it was as if, over time, I had become accustomed to receiving the *symbolic vesture* of a nurturing mother (as well as all the terrifying *vestures* that she had summoned me to assume), making it easier for me to experience her sessions with a certain tranquillity, within the realms of possibility.

The main thing in a treatment like this would be for the patient to survive her attacks and to keep "chewing" the terror she projected in the sessions, in order to return something psychically "nourishing". It was necessary to accept her "psychic absences" because, in fact, her psyche was often taken to a "non-place", a non-existence. Realising that she was sleeping in order to be veiled and protected under my gaze seemed to me the best thing I could do in those moments.

After three years of treatment, when she had managed to start the master's degree she wanted and was showing more and more vivacity and an attenuation of her symptoms – even though they were increasingly accentuating her marital conflicts[34] – the analysand stopped treatment. She didn't take well to the idea that I would be moving my consulting room to another space (even though it was in the same building and on the same floor), even though I had brought up the subject of the move well in advance. She said that she was very fond of that consulting room, that she would not adapt to the new one, and that she felt very grateful since I had helped her greatly, but that she wished to bring the treatment to an end. I tried to interpret her fear of change, of the new, and her fantasy of hostility towards the new place, but it didn't have the desired effect, and she actually ended the treatment.

The case reported ended in a negative therapeutic reaction. Unfortunately, we can't always escape it. However, the selected section (which leaves out a lot of relevant information) is a way of trying to exemplify the importance of the couch in illnesses beyond neurosis. **The couch is the instrument that facilitates the emergence of the analysand's *cloud state* and enables the installation of the *shared cloud state* (a third space of interlocution between the internal spaces of each member of the analytic pair). More than this, it allows for the experience and re-experience of situations that could not be reached face-to-face. It was necessary to tolerate the mixture of autistic absences[35] and the attacks the analysand directed at me, so that she could succeed in *re-forming* herself through her analysis. The couch afforded her the possibility of enacting "psychic absence" in a accompanied way, libidinising the scene of internal absence played out in the session for the purpose of working it through.** There isn't a specific speech or scene that I could select to exemplify the process. In this case, part of the technique ended up being to tolerate and respect her moments of absence, of a great "blank", a great "void", so that she could feel accepted and respected as she is – to create and *re-form* herself from this "blank". The more she felt respected, feeling that the space of analysis was welcoming to her suffering, the less her autistic absence came into play (periods of incommunicado time when she didn't say anything, nor did she respond to any word I might say – which, when I realised, still at the beginning, led me simply to respect her internal time).

Only the couch could provide this analysis. Not only was it fundamental for the analysand, it was also fundamental for me. My exhaustion and my facial reaction to her attacks, especially the first ones, would influence her continuity. It is "easier" to endure transferential attacks with the guarantee of experiencing them minimally in private, without the analysand's "attacking" psyche measuring the analyst's facial reactions. Sometimes analysands carry out sadistic attacks and, depending on the case, perverse attacks, which would depend on seeing the analyst's face/reaction in order to be completely satisfied. The couch also serves here as an object that forces the symptom or disorder to seek third pathways, rather than a direct route to the analyst-object, just as it protects the session from turning into an "ordinary conversation". Its presence and use reaffirms and assures everyone: "we are working from the transferential virtuality". Working on the couch helps the analysand to understand, albeit *a posteriori*, that the intensities deposited transferentially onto the figure of the analyst are part of their psychic illness. Work on the couch helps the analyst to receive the transference and the symbolic vestures that the analysand covers them with, protecting the quality of their listening and intervention.

If we intend to work as deeply as possible in an analysis, it is important that the analyst feels a minimal degree of comfort in order to do so. As Freud explained, the analysand's massive gaze in a face-to-face situation hinders the necessary immersion into the cloud state that analytic work requires.

Ogden reinforces this position by stating that both members of the pair (analyst/analysand) need a minimally private space in order for the intimate shared space to come into being.

In predominantly non-neurotic cases, the analysand often does not know what it is to have their psychic privacy respected. Thus, their initial reaction – if they have not experienced such privacy in the constitution of their psyche – will likely be to resist the idea of lying on the couch. They do not know the notion of privacy, only that of invasion, and so they preconceive the couch as something invasive, since within them there is no representation of what it would mean to experience privacy. Yet it seems to me possible to indicate its use, provided its function for the joint work is made clear. In such cases, privacy itself becomes something new to be lived – something that contributes to the process of *re-formation* in analysis.

If we are speaking of creating a support for the analysand's psychic development, we must understand the importance of doing so through "something" that symbolises a third space – the *couch/diwan*[36] – a metaphorical space, an object of support that can be taken as a depository of the analysand's internalities, just as a toy is in a child's analysis. The analysand's psychic support cannot be the analyst's concrete gaze: this idea, as well as damaging the analyst's ability to listen and intervene,[37] would take the treatment into the realm of superficiality.

In a face-to-face modality, even if it is not their intention, the analyst is placed in a role that involves "approving" the analysand's desperate search for every one of their movements, as if serving as a kind of support for their existence. The analysand will seek "approval" from every move the analyst makes and will feel persecuted or "disapproved" when they don't find it. Obviously, we need to keep the analysand supported, but by shifting this support to the couch, as a third object, which mediates the transference, which delimits spaces: "You exist, I exist, and there is a third space of exchange".

The indication of the couch also serves as the introduction of a space for play, which is not a simple projection and massive introjection in a concretely scopic transference towards the analyst. Understanding the couch as an object open to the malleability of play, to the malleability of the *cloud state*, containing in it all the facets we explored in Part I of this book, added to all that has been exposed in Part II, has gradually led me, over the years, to indicate the couch for all the clinical cases, so far, that came my way.[38] For predominantly neurotic cases, face-to-face care would even end up being a waste of the treatment's potential – something like asking a whale to swim in the shallows.

If we understand the couch as a mother/analyst body-object,[39] as Winnicott theorised, or even as a generational space, like a womb, as we saw in Bollas, or from other authorial positions that try the same vertex in other ways, we understand that the couch helps to create the separation between the I and the not-I, a boundary that appears blurred in the most severe suffering. It seems to me mistaken to think that the couch would leave the analysand alone. We are right behind them, they feel our physical presence, and this resonates transferentially in the work of the analytic pair. The couch must not serve an impossible neutrality[40] or the installation of mortifying silences. The analyst's psyche is always influencing the session, whether they want it to or not. There's no escaping this idea, because even silence is a psychic communication from the analyst.

In this sense, in "mortifying" moments of an analysis, the constant voice of the analyst, as a kind of rhythmic soothing, becomes fundamental in the management of the treatments on the couch. I'm not gradually reinforcing the necessary nature of playing for nothing. **The analyst needs to "play" with the psychic materials brought to the session by the analysand, entering into the modality of work that Roussillon defined, inspired by Winnicott's squiggle game,**

as *psychoanalytic conversation*.[41] **Therefore, it is necessary to approach the virtuality of the transference as the stage onto which the *cloud state* – what is presented of the analysand's psychic life – is projected. We must "play" and intervene in this world according to what the analysand's psyche "asks for"**, much as we would intervene in the play offered by a child analysand during a session. For example, in the clinical section I explained earlier, I fulfilled the role that the analysand's transference play placed me in: that of the nurturing mother (among other types of roles that have been exemplified). Sometimes these roles are more silent and implicit; at other times, they depend more on the active presence of the analyst's voice, like the Winnicottian squiggle game – when the analyst adds an association to connect with the analysand's, weaving a long thread together, always interlaced with his theoretical-clinical thought, but also with his reverie and his countertransference.

The analyst should not place himself merely as an observer outside the scene, as one who might occasionally make a remark, not least because such a position is illusory. Such an attempt to place themselves outside the scene is, in itself, a way of being in the scene, of occupying it through an absence. In general, in predominantly non-neurotic illnesses, the frequency of the analyst's speech (analogous to the aforementioned squiggle game) needs to be much higher than in a classic analysis, helping to weave the plot. **The analyst's speech is not "surgical". The analyst's speech sets out to "play" and offer plasticity to the contents *that* emerge from the analysand's *cloud state*.** The analyst must be immersed in the field of play, just as a child analyst is, and this forces him to develop his malleability. It's a question of the analyst "scribbling" sentences together with the analysand in order to weave together the fabric of a psychic body without borders, when this is the case.

The issue of malleability is fundamental and must be made explicit. The indication of the couch needs to be explained to the analysand in such a way that they can minimally understand its function. It must be made clear, with or without words, that working on the couch does not require the analysand to submit to the analyst's method. Rather, the indication of the couch involves an invitation to trust the analyst with whatever comes and goes, based on working together. Just as Ogden indicates the couch by justifying each person's privacy, I believe we should "justify" our indication by taking into account the particularities of each case.

For didactic purposes, I'll try to outline here how I usually indicate the couch. In the following example, I ended up creating a "big statement", but in reality, the writing only serves as an example of the varied possibilities, depending on the uniqueness of each analysand, and, because of this, it would certainly have to be adapted, taking into account what was worked on together during the evaluation period.[42] The example could be:

"After we've gone through this period of joint evaluation, discussed your desire to continue working, discussed the fees and thought about the ideal frequency for our meetings, it would be interesting if, from now on, we started working with the couch. I realise that you often worry about my reactions, about what I might think of what you say; you worry that I understand you; and perhaps sometimes you are more attentive to what I will say or how I will react to what you tell me. You don't have to worry about this, you can be sure that I'll be connected to what you bring me, even if you don't see me when you're on the couch. Moreover, I feel that I can listen to you more deeply and even help you more profoundly without looking at you directly. Part of my work is to allow what you tell me to carry my thoughts into the necessary depths, and, strange though it may seem to you, I am able to do this better while looking at the wall, at the bookshelf, the empty armchair in front of me, or at the clouds outside the window … You might find me amusing for saying this, 'These psychoanalysts are peculiar'. [I would add, perhaps, some small joke about my work that made sense in the light of what had been built together during the assessment sessions.] I will be here with you for whatever may come, so please feel at ease here. We are only beginning a journey together. You can be sincere with me. There may be moments when you feel you love me, but you may also feel a great deal of hatred – even to the point of wanting to swear at me, should that occur. Just, please, don't hit me![43] [I would add, good-humouredly, authorising at the same time the movement of humour and of the aggressive and destructive aspects of the self within the session, while also setting a limit to such destruction.] I'll be here with you, and you'll feel my presence; there's no need to worry about me. Whenever I'm silent, you can be sure that I'm accompanying you with my thoughts, and nothing prevents you from turning your head and peeking at me, should that seem a good idea. Lying on the couch, I believe you will feel just as free to give yourself over to your thoughts as I do, and we will think and feel together whatever may arise for you as you lie there."

This fictitious referral to the couch tries to contemplate different aspects of a psychic life. It should also be borne in mind that, in session, unlike the written text, I would emphasise a colloquiality linked to everyday life. Obviously, some parts of this idea could be selected for one analysand, others for another … saying less for one, more for another. For some, far fewer words; for others, something else that the example doesn't cover. It all depends on what you hear and build up during the initial evaluation period. The fact is: whatever I say, I always tend to convey calmness in my tone of voice, coupled with a few doses of humour (provided this is not forced, but genuine).

Resistance is always hostility towards the analyst. I play with the extreme (the analysand hitting me, throwing me out of the window, or something of the sort) in order to authorise them to bring out things in the future that they imagine could attack me. This kind of intervention goes some way towards marking out the space of the session as different from ordinary social relationships, where aggression is not usually welcomed. This analytical position will authorise them to work on their oedipal hostility, but also on a possible trauma stemming from their primary narcissism, a possible complaint about not having been properly welcomed in their early life.

It is essential that the analyst ensures they survive whatever may come, and I say this while pointing out that we can play with hostility. We can play at destroying, just as some children in analysis need to destroy a little toy figure. We can play at taking ourselves apart. We can even say this, in words that are intelligible to the analysand, if it seems interesting for the treatment, but the limit is set. Our subtext would imply something like: "You can use your sessions in any way that suits you, as long as we don't destroy ourselves beyond the virtuality of the transference." This kind of statement simultaneously speaks to the playful dimension of the analytic process – which I believe we must never overlook – and establishes limits and boundaries. The "play" ends if the physical integrity of the analysand or the analyst is at risk. Certainly, other enunciations, when the couch is indicated, can or should be more emphasised or less emphasised. This example has endeavoured to elucidate the work with destructiveness and to demonstrate the double path that an enunciation can take.[44]

The use of the couch alludes to the presence-absence paradox, based on a subjective gaze – as opposed to a concrete gaze. The analyst is always marking their presence in some way, whether through their breathing or through any bodily movement they make in their armchair, just as they also mark their presence through the constancy of their voice, exercised by the *psychoanalytic conversation* (this association-play, like the game of doodling). From an auditory perspective, the analysand can always be sure of the analyst's presence. On the couch, the analysand will experience the paradox of being both alone and accompanied, based on the constancy of the sessions, and will incessantly disassemble and reassemble themselves in the eternal process of *re-formation.*

The couch, in this line of understanding, beyond being the *instrumentum princeps* for the analysis of neuroses and for the classical model, proves to be the best channel through which the most precarious *psychic regions* may emerge and be worked through. In any treatment, we are always dealing with the analysand's psychic life as a whole. Thus, a session may unfold on the basis of neurotic manifestations until, at a certain point, something of another order may emerge.

22.4 The consulting room as a whole and its connection to unconscious processes

Once again, it's important to emphasise the etymological aspect of the *couch/diwan* as a meeting room of the utmost importance and, from this, to also reflect on the other objects that make up this room, beyond the couch itself. The psychoanalytic reflection of Bollas[45] would lead us to say that every choice – including architectural ones, the design of interiors, whatever they may be – is connected with our unconscious movements and with our self. To perceive/listen to this is of the utmost importance, since accessing our own unconscious choices has repercussions for a better listening. Let us not forget that Freud insisted on arranging his ancient artefacts in his consulting room, and it does not seem possible to me to regard them as mere decoration; rather, they are material objects that represent his archaeological model within the analytic room, intimately bound to the proposal of thinking about the couch and the work based on it under the prism of reminiscences.[46] Based on Bollas's thinking, we should recognise an unconscious meaning in these environmental architectural arrangements – propositions that reaffirm the inexistence of a supposedly aseptic neutrality in the space of psychoanalytic care. The analyst is abstinent, but is always offering potential objects of use. By way of analogy, let us remember that, from the very first session with a child, the analyst visually offers toys and possibilities of play in the session. In this sense, the analyst would be offering the consulting room and its component objects so that they might possibly be taken up as objects of use for unconscious communications – just as he offers his psyche to the analytic work.

The analyst's room and, above all, the couch *communicate* something and become objects available for use during analysis. In the analytic posture, the analyst remains abstinent, but believing oneself to be neutral is an unattainable ideal and, more than that, a denial, as it fails to recognise the relationship between the analyst's Unconscious and the objects they have chosen to compose their *setting*. According to Bollas, objects evoke much more than representations: they evoke procedures, movements, transformations that, ultimately, are at least auxiliary to the analyst. It seems honest and transparent to recognise that we manifest our *self* in some way through the way we compose the interior of our consulting room (*diwan*). Therefore, the analyst is always offering psychic material to the analysand, even when the analyst remains completely silent.

The idea that the analyst is always offering potential psychic material to converse with the analysand's *cloud state*, even if unintentionally, is also important when thinking about the indication of the couch. In a face-to-face treatment, the analyst is *presenting* their facial expressions to be taken by the analysand as components of their transferential relationship. So again, when we indicate the use of the couch, we are offering something other than the concreteness of our gaze. Based on the postulation of the *couch in latency* and the developments that surround it, Roussillon points out the importance of the couch as a representative of the analytical process,[47] at least of what the analyst has experienced as an analysand. Would it not be important to reflect that all the objects that make up the analytic room – the Turkish-Ottoman *couch/diwan* – are offered for the analysand's psychic use? The graphic materials and toys we offer for use in child analysis would be the most obvious examples to correlate with this proposal.

I realise that, just as the analyst's psyche is offered to transferential work, so are all the other objects that make up the room, including the inanimate ones. Let's say, for example, that we're talking about a desk, blank papers with the potential to be written on, psychoanalysis books (repositories of knowledge) on the shelf … The analysand won't necessarily make psychic use of these elements in the same way as the analyst (who chose them to make up the room, albeit unconsciously). Nor is this even desirable, though it may be possible. Yet some kind of relation is established, whether "beneficial" or not. I believe it is of value for each analyst to reflect upon the inanimate objects that compose his consulting room. Paintings, photographs of Freud, books on psychoanalysis, when present in the analytic room, play a role in supporting the analyst's listening, just as Roussillon's *couch in latency* assures his relation with his own listening, and they are, in a way, a kind of totem[48] (psychoanalytic ancestors, guardians of analytic practice).

It is certainly no coincidence that in my *consulting room/diwan* I keep shelves with books on psychoanalysis and, above all, of poetry; or even that I choose (out of pure aesthetic whim on my part, but certainly influenced by the model of thinking about the clinic that I have been presenting) to position the couch-furniture towards a window with a view of the clouds.[49] All architectural features make themselves present and may have varied functions in the analytic process. Such objects form part of the *diwan* as a room of important meetings, and fulfil auxiliary roles (at least for the analyst's listening), just as much as the couch-furniture (in the sense of what Roussillon postulated with regard to the *couch in latency*) – though not in the way Bollas theorised evocative objects.[50]

I believe that all psychoanalysts are familiar with a situation in which the analysand comments on a certain object in the consulting room, be it a painting, a book or some other element. The analyst has chosen them, even if unconsciously, as elements to be offered for the psychic use of their analysands – as usable objects, much like toys are for children. If we take Christopher Bollas's thinking, the objects of the external world are capable of becoming transformational objects for the development of the *self*. That is, they can be taken as transformative elements by the analysand, since, for Bollas, we seek not only repetition, but also the new and transformation through object relations – whether through human relations or through inanimate objects. Any production – for example, some music the analysand happens to listen to – may become an object of use in session. In an analytic environment, objects (including the analyst) are potentially offered for transformational use, whether or not the analyst has previously reflected on this.

We could also use an example that goes beyond the space of the session, but is linked to the transferential relationship: an analysand, for a certain period, began to take magazines from the waiting room to read at home and eventually even stole some, without ever accusing herself (in fact, without final proof, it may not have been her, but everything leads me to believe that it was). It took me a while to realise her practice, which she understood as natural ("I always understood that the magazines were there to be read and I often preferred to read them at home", she told me).[51] It is not the point here to discuss whether her reasons were envious, or whether she was seeking to take with her "something good" from the analyst – that is, contents and internal states of the analyst which would reinforce, within herself, aspects worked through in session, in the transference, or all of these together. The fact is that, for this analysand, the magazines in the waiting room were materials that formed part of her analysis and of her transferential relationship with me. Not so different from this is the research via Google (or other online means) that analysands carry out before starting an analysis, or even during it, in search of information about the analyst.

Both what's on the internet about the analyst and the way they set up their consulting room are part of the public and manifest realm of us, the analysts. All the objects on offer contain traces of our most intimate *psychic regions* and are indeed sought out by analysands from the perspective of the object relationship. A good number of my analysands even know the football team I support, because of Google searches. These analysands have told me that, before they even had their first session with me, they accessed a piece of material in which I was interviewed as a writer about my creative process, in which I reported that I liked to start the day by finding out about the football club I support.

This reveals that even the most neurotic analysand seeks the "concreteness" of their analyst, who becomes session material sooner or later. In this case, the club of the analyst's heart becomes material for working on issues related to identification (when the analysand supports the same club) or rivalry (when they support a rival club).[52] This example is interesting because we're talking about internal issues projected onto a third space and culture. It's not interesting that this type of psychic demand for "investigation" occurs from the concrete gaze of the analyst's facial expressions in a treatment. There is always a thirst in the analysand for the person of the analyst, and a curiosity about what they might be thinking regarding the psychic material expressed in session.

What, then, are we to say about those analysands, themselves psychoanalysts, who come to know aspects of the analyst's private life by sharing the same environment – the psychoanalytic community – and who seek "factual" information by such means? The desire to glimpse the title of a book resting in the consulting room is but a concrete way for the analysand to try to relate more intimately to the analyst; yet, because this is a third object, the speculation around it becomes somewhat more interesting to "play with" in the analysis than the concrete speculation of the face-to-face gaze.

In this respect, the speculation of the analysand lying down and facing a white wall, or the movement of the clouds in the window and the forms that may be projected there, is richer than projection based on the concreteness of the analyst's gaze – regardless of which *psychic regions* of the analysand predominate in the analytic work.

Beyond the analysand, it's interesting to think about the analyst's relationship with the composition of his room/*diwan*. The analyst will live with these objects for hours, days, years, while listening to his analysands, and these objects also come to function as evocative objects of great force within the analyst. It seems to me important that the analyst relate to these objects in a playful and poetic way, and that they serve as facilitators of the analyst's *cloud state*, since they are evocative of their *internal regions*, of their analytical working self.

It is to these objects that your gaze will be turned most of the time during your treatment, and their playful and poetic function, contained in your *analytical cloud state*, can be indispensable to your psychic work during analyses, especially in clinical situations where we would be dealing with arid or excessively sick psyches. The human being and their *creational* potential par excellence end up involuntarily creating totems of reference. For some analysts (perhaps even in a problematic way), figures of Freud's persona occupy a place similar to that of Jesus Christ or Muhammad, as a kind of religion, which inevitably also leads to blindness.

Let's not forget that *couch/diwan*[53] originally (and literally), through its Persian lineage, signifies a poetic work, the volume that gathers together a poetic oeuvre; and Freud makes clear in his work his appreciation for poets and for poetic-making. From this perspective, the poetic is part of analysis – not only in Freud's thought or in his writings. The *diwan*, its etymology, alludes to and contains the analytical process, regardless of Freud's conscious thinking about the use of the couch. We gain nothing by crediting chance or randomness with the fact that Freud became attached to it as an essential instrument of his practice, or that it is *nonsensical* to reflect on the objects that make up the important analytic meeting room (*diwan*) and are always, in some way, offered to the analysand as objects of use. **The analyst's every move in session presupposes choices, even if they are unconscious. My understanding is that the analyst's psyche also places itself in a *cloud state*, as a creative procedural function of the *creational* order (to influence and assist in the composition of the analytical transferential field), during the session (and this includes the objects present in their consulting room). The psychoanalytic work would take place in the encounter, in the third space, which encompasses the clouds of analyst and analysand.**

22.5 Considerations on child analysis – the couch as bed, boat and castle

Although the couch has been linked to the analysis of adults since the beginning, it is interesting to discuss it from the point of view of analysing children.[54] If Klein[55] thought of the analysis of children from the point of view of how the couch was used as an auxiliary/facilitating object in the analysis of adults, let's create the opposite path: analysis of children as a theoretical-clinical basis for thinking about the analysis of adults.

In analyses with children, the couch usually performs functions that are just as important as in analyses with adults, even though it is naturally not used in its classic form. For them, the couch can fulfil an essential role, even if implicitly.[56] Children play with the couch, they bring it into the narrative they are constructing. It is evoked as a useful element in their fantasies and seen as a potential object of use, with an omnipotent *creational* function that aids unconscious communication. Children make the couch into a bed, a boat, a bedroom, a castle and/or any demarcation of space that suits them ... in fact, the couch can be anything in the child's play. In many cases, the analysis room itself is perceived by them as a bedroom and/or as the analyst's house and/or as a continuation of their own house/room. Curiously, these subjective attitudes of the child are reminiscent of the Turkish-Ottoman etymological aspect of *couch/diwan*: a meeting room of the highest importance.

Placing the analysis room in the spectrum of a "make-believe", like a house/bedroom – or the couch as a bed – is nothing more than an approximation, in terms of familiarity, with the psychic material of those children who, in fact, come to the session precisely because of conflicts that arise from the family environment, from home.

It is essential that the analysis room can be a "receptive house". On the other hand, the couch as a "bed", when not dealing with issues of abuse, could allude to what André Green theorises about the classical method as a model of the dream. The child somehow knows, even if they are not fully aware of it, that there is no censorship in the dream. When they fall asleep, their desires, fears and traumas circulate and erupt in a way that doesn't happen in waking life.

To some degree, even if it's minimal (let's not compare it to an adult, of course), something in the culture and the family environment restricts the fulfilment of their impulses, and that's what I'm talking about. Castration (not being able to do everything) kicks in as soon as you leave your mother's womb, starting with the impossibility of returning to the protection of the womb. Right from the start, the baby has to deal with not being completely satisfied. Total satisfaction is illusory, even for a sufficiently well-supported child.

The presence of a "bed" (couch) in the treatment room signals to the children, even unconsciously, that their inner issues can emerge uncensored. In this way, we know that the concrete presence of furniture facilitates the emergence of Oedipal content, such as nocturnal enuresis. **The infantile dimension activates the *couch/diwan* into a *cloud state*. The child's developing *psychic regions* offer psychoanalytic work even greater plasticity compared to the *standard* adult sessions. The objects in the analysis room (and the analyst too, of course) are**

taken by the children in all their power and re-vested in *symbolic vesture*, serving as ancillary forms to their unconscious manifestations. The entire analyst's room, and the whole range of toys and graphic materials offered in the consulting room, are embraced in its playful malleability.

Even when analysing adults, we work with the child who lives within them, Sándor Ferenczi would point out.[57] Working to relate to the child who lives "inside" each analysand would confer an intention to access the primal functioning of the psyche. In this conception, we would be working directly with Freud's child-poet, Winnicott's child who creates the world and Bollas's child who seeks the transformational object, exploring the poetic facet of the *diwan*.

Marion Milner reports, in the text *An Adult Patient Uses Toys*,[58] that an adult analysand, on learning that her analyst worked with children, asked her to offer the materials used by them in analysis – in this case, drawing sheets. Her analysand would be a "serious case" (with whom electroconvulsive therapy was necessary) and, we could say, took the possibility of developing her inner world through the blank sheet of paper, a circumscribed space – metaphorically, too, this blank space would be a potential and malleable space, in which she would have the freedom to experiment, to make a mess, and, above all, to play and to exist. Working with sculpture, painting, drawing and all forms of play and theatre are correlated with the idea of thinking about the *couch/diwan* from the point of view of etymology, since these forms of work "embody" the function of "cloud play", the malleability of play, contained in the *diwan*. It is from this listening perspective that the analyses of children and of adults resemble each other.

The line that separates child analysis from adult analysis can be a tenuous one. Let's remember, as stated in Part I, Chapter 4, "The couch, the child who lives in the adult, and the technical daring of Sándor Ferenczi", Ferenczi's account of an adult analysand who hugged him, called him grandpa and spoke to him as if he really were.

This staging only alludes, in a more concrete way, to what has been described about a transferential *symbolic vesture* being placed on the analyst, arising from the *cloud state of* the session.

What seems essential to underline, with regard to the examples cited, is that the theoretical-clinical reflections of Milner and Ferenczi were not intended to defend the abandonment of the couch in favour of a face-to-face treatment (even though, of course, the situations recounted included an exchange of glances between analyst and analysand during the session), but rather to contemplate the play of the child who lives within the adult. In other words, thinking about the child who lives within the adult is thinking from the inside out, whereas primarily defending face-to-face could be a way of thinking from the outside in. Psychoanalytic work with children is based on the malleability with which they *re-vest*, from their internal world, each "concrete" object in the psychoanalytic session – a malleability that is also essential for thinking about the analysis of adults.

22.6 Sharing singular inner poetry and the presentation of symbolic vesture – penultimate words

"I am on the verge of being shared / I adjust the clouds in the eye", say the verses by Manoel de Barros.[59] Let's not reduce the intention of his verses to psychoanalytical interpretations (which always diminish the amplitude of poetic thought), but let's take them as a stimulus and allow ourselves to think/play with some of the countless possibilities of relating to this artistic fragment. Do Manoel de Barros' verses emphasise the importance of play? Are they talking about the paradox between inside and outside of oneself? Do his verses place the clouds as a stage for the projection of what is being shared? Is he explicitly talking about making public (in book form) what is private? If we think in psychoanalytical terms, we can take these verses as inspiration for a discussion on what the analysand shares with the analyst in session.

Such an idea would be that the clouds contain the poet's play, but are also the place where he projects such play, as if to say: "I shall share my innermost being through the clouds; pay attention to them, for with them I shall play, and from them my depth shall arise." Manoel de Barros' verses can also lead us to further questions: in an analysis session, where is it interesting to look? Where is the stage for the staging of the Unconscious, the parade of *symbolic vesture* and the malleable possibility of changing them? Quite possibly, the stage would be the consulting room and its atmosphere as a whole. The scenes of the stage are never self-sufficient; it is always through interaction with them that art is created – and the same can be said of analysis.

It's difficult to read your own internal book through the eyes of others. An analysis is carried out on the basis of what can be seen in the movement of its clouds, in the play of its internal clouds. It's a matter of "looking at the movements within", from the *symbolic vesture* woven on the stage of the session/*diwan*.

The malleability contained in this premise translates into making use of the ability to figure like a toy in an analysis session, because it is always the *Darstellung* (presentation/figuration/dramatising) that is the agent of the psychoanalytic session. The representation (ideational content) is there within the Unconscious, it is "untouchable": we try to grasp for it through derivatives, through the *symbolic vesture* that cover them. The content of the cloud is water; the Unconscious is deep water. The condensation of the cloud weaves the *symbolic vesture*.

During an analysis session, the analyst can be used figuratively by the analysand, through the transference, in a certain form, and within a few seconds the form is already different. To think of a simple example, let's say that the analyst is being taken, in some enunciation by the analysand, as a father (or rather, in the *symbolic vesture* of a father), and within 10 seconds they are already being used, transferentially, in another form, another *vesture*.

The analysand "places" upon the analyst a *symbolische Verkleidung*, a symbolic vesture. The analysand puts one on, removes it, dons another, and lives in constant change of costumes upon the analyst. More precisely still, the analysand does this with all the elements of the session: they take both the analyst and the *couch/diwan* as an amorphous mass, and mould them as they "want" (internally need) them to look. All this is done unconsciously, within the transferential relation they establish.

Taking what happens on the *couch/diwan* as *a cloud state* allows us to "float", as Freud's technique indicates, but at the same time this notion makes it clear to the psychoanalyst that floating is, in fact, extremely difficult. It would be frivolous and simplistic for the psychoanalyst to think that they have spent an entire session, perhaps months or years, tied to just one or two figures/roles or a pair of transferential modes.

The cloud state "draws water" from the *internal regions* and provides the malleable space of play, but at the same time it mercilessly marks the castration of the analyst. When they get used to the transferential figuration that the analysand supposedly confers on them, they need to be aware that the wind (the analysand's associations) can blow in such a way that, for a while, the analyst will be transferentially amorphous, until they turn into another form, apparently disconnected from the one they have just become accustomed to. Feeling amorphous (in the transferential field) can be distressing for the analyst. It is necessary to be amorphous for a while, until the analysand "sees" (re-vests) the analyst in a new *symbolic vesture* in the transferential scene – in the waiting time in the transition of scenes, just like in the theatre, when this moment is literally marked by the effect of a smoke machine, which creates a "big cloud" to blur and obscure the audience's vision, until a new scene materialises.

The Chilean poet Pablo Neruda named his writing chair *La nube* (the cloud). Following our propositions, we could play with the idea that the *cloud state* "projected" itself onto his armchair, or invested libidinally, in Freudian terms, in his armchair. From the moment the armchair becomes *La nube*, a special armchair for writing, it is no longer just any armchair, it is loaded and "lined" with the playful and poetic malleability of clouds. It's about thinking of the couch in this way. From the moment it is invested, cathexised, in session, it ceases to be just any object. The couch "proper" (concrete furniture) and the analysis room as a whole serve the *cloud state* that *presents* itself in the analytical work.

Transference and all its derivatives would also be nothing more and nothing less than condensations of the "source water of the Unconscious". In the early days, in *The Interpretation of Dreams*,[60] for example, Freud used the term *transference/Übertragung*[61] also within the context of the mechanisms surrounding the dream. His primary conception is that of transposing into one figure what is originally from another. We're talking about wearing a costume, just like in the theatre. This is what presents itself in the field of analysis, dreams and symptoms, and what Freud called a "false connection".[62]

From the perspective we are adopting, we could say: "what we have direct access to are the symbolic vestures (which veil the true representation), and it is only through these that we can attempt to set in motion the contents residing in the Unconscious". Freud makes it clear, throughout his work, that it is through such derivatives that psychoanalytic work may be done.

The *couch/diwan* is the body, the poetry, the customs-house (*aduana*) and the important meeting room that defines directions. It is noteworthy that I "condense" what I theorise about the metaphor of the *cloud* and the *couch/diwan*, for this is precisely the point to raise: *to think of the work on the couch/diwan as cloud* (a third space materialising the encounter between the cloud of the analyst and that of the analysand), in what it aids the internal movement and in what remains latent within it.

Let's not forget that lying on the couch would still provide the primal corporeal-object support present in the theorisations of Winnicott, Bollas and other authors presented in the book. Not looking directly at the analyst doesn't mean not sensitively feeling their presence, their body, their breathing and their words. The *couch/diwan* is this embryonic field of each person's poetry, accompanied by the analyst.

The cloud is the depository of desire that creates forms, contours. Part of the analytic work is to plunge into the *cloud state* until one feels within it, to lie down in it. It is the potential form-non-form, in which paradox coexists. The cloud-cotton serves as the weaving of the scenic costumes – it can be taken, to a certain extent, as a *creational* engine, if we follow in the footsteps of Pontalis, Bollas, Winnicott and Bion, understanding that to lie on the couch-cloud is also to lie in the womb that generates, to transport oneself to other scenes, lived or to be lived, infinitely, in beneficial or malefic forms. The cloud makes monsters and gods appear, it can split into a thousand, tear itself apart, contain many images in one, contain several that interconnect or not. Being-non-being. The cloud lends itself to the *creational* required for *re-form*. It creates the rain that washes, that torments, that bathes and gives life, that strikes with lightning. It contains electricity and light, but it can also contain darkness. It converses with the rainbow and can accompany our desire or challenge us. It may be stubborn, evade desire, contradict us; but it may also seduce us. It can be the father, the mother, a hug, anger, love, the analyst. On a transferential level, it can be "everything". "To describe the clouds I would have to be very fast; in a fraction of a second they cease to be these and become others", as the verses of Wisława Szymborska (2011) say. For the analyst, who also works with historicisation and seeks to construct or deconstruct the significations that dwell within their analysands, this metaphor may serve as an additional auxiliary tool.

The psychoanalyst works with psychic "matter". To be a psychoanalyst (etymologically, one who decomposes or participates in the decomposition of what is in the psychic field) is also to be a "psycho-artisan" (one who composes or participates in the composition of what is in the psychic field).[63] The psychoanalyst is one who works with and upon psychic "matter" in an artisanal and singular way, not just in its decomposition.

It is essential in our work to think about the eternal process of composition and decomposition present in the "cloud play" of the session. The cloud "itself", which we see outside in the sky, is also a kind of mirror. In the psychoanalytic process, it's about looking at oneself, accompanied by another human being (the analyst), but not necessarily moulded by that human being's gaze; without making analysis an alienation from the desiring gaze of the other, as Lacan might point out.

The *couch/diwan-cloud* is a *virtual stage* and therefore lives from the condensations of all the *psychic regions*. If we take the first Freudian topic as an aid to this thought, it's *as if* the barriers of the topic were asleep. However, it is *as if* in its virtuality, the *cloud* being the terrain of *presentation* that would include the dream, the symptom, the transference and any other form of *presentification*. Freud[64] cites his influence on G. T. Fechner and his proposition of a "dream stage" to think about a psychic locality, and to begin theorising and presenting his first topic to us.

There is a virtuality in the transference play. It is experienced *as if it* were real, and, to a certain extent, it is. The transference is not a psychosis, it's an *as if*, in the sense of playing out a fantasy, a narrative, delegating roles to oneself and the analyst, moulding situations – unconsciously.

It´s important to realise that the proposal here is to offer different angles of looking at a stimulus-proposition, in order to reflect on the psychoanalytic process and on inner functioning. "Multilingualism is the target",[65] **the cloud is the space where all the internal regional languages can converse (or not). The *cloud* "gathers" what evaporates from the *psychic regions* and *manifests/presents* it formally.**

When we treat neurosis, we are always "touching" the figuration-staging, in the sense that this is what we are able to access. This *presentation* is what assists us in working with what is otherwise inaccessible. It is this that "converses" with representation (ideational content), so as to resolve the internal conflict. It is the "direction" and interpretation that we give to the scene and its *vestures* that may mobilise the deepest internalities. Our role is also to organise the scenes and roles that the analysand transposes into the analysis without knowing, on a conscious level, what they are dramatising.

When we think of "non-neuroses", if we can speak more generally, the analyst would be called upon to offer the potential capacity of their *creational* psychic processes in order to help the analysand weave *symbolic vesture* to "cover" the nakedness and rawness of their wounds exposed to the incessant cold of the traumatic. **In these cases, one of the analyst's roles would be to offer their psychic resources as a weaving capacity, either to help weave representations where there are none, or to *weave/sew/re-form* the *self*, or even to remove "false garments" (which don't warm affectively) that would cover up an underdeveloped *self*. There would have to be an *exchange/re-formation* of skin, via weaving. Ultimately, it's a matter of the analyst conducting the session into the allegorical dimension of internal malleable play.**

The *cloud state* is both a weaving workshop and an incarnation of the *Darstellung* in the analysis room (if we take Roussillon's idea of incarnation mentioned earlier). Its movement alludes to the mechanisms of displacement and condensation, and within it lies the character of elevation present in Freud's proposal of sublimation. Its restless, mobile quality also figures the life of the drives and even the motor pole (if we think in Freud's metapsychology). Returning to the clouds of childhood, from within, allows for an elasticity of gaze that is outward ("to see the world better"), but at the same time is inward looking.

The metaphor of clouds serves as an auxiliary means for understanding the transferences that must be – and indeed are – established for the analytic process to take place. It is the embodiment of the "as if", which alludes to the transference to the analyst "as father", "as mother", "as brother", "as good", "as bad", or as any other transferential mode that needs to operate in analysis. It's clear, however, that thinking of the psychoanalytic session from this perspective depends on the psychoanalyst's good management, as in any other technical use. The analysand not seeing the analyst directly, as in the face-to-face modality, doesn't mean that they won't feel their presence, their body, their breathing and their words. The *couch/diwan* is this embryonic field of each person's poetry, accompanied by the analyst.

Percy Shelley (1792–1822), one of England's greatest poets, offers us glimpses that he could well have been a psychoanalyst, only corroborating Freud's thought that the wisdom of poets nourished the very foundations of psychoanalysis. In the passage I present below, Shelley appears as an ally to the psychoanalytic theoretical-clinical thought we are working through, and seems almost to summarise, in a single paragraph, our work as psychoanalysts – interrogating poetry and its function even against "the recurrence of impressions blunted by repetition."

> ... poetry defeats the curse that binds us, subject to the accident of the impressions that surround us. And if it extends its figurative curtain or pulls back the dark veil life from the scene of things, it also creates, for us, a being within our being. It makes us the inhabitants of a world in which the familiar world is chaos. It reproduces the common universe of which we are inhabitants and are aware, and expels from our inner vision the film of

> familiarity that obscures the wonder of our being. Poetry compels us to feel what we perceive and to imagine what we know. It creates a new universe after it has been annihilated in our minds by the recurrence of loving impressions woven by repetition. Poetry justifies Tasso's courageous and true words: "Non merita nome di criatore, se non Iddio ed il Poeta."[66]

It wouldn't be interesting to decompose or reduce Shelley's already lucid and poetic statement; even so, let's translate his quote from Tasso: "He does not deserve the name of creator, but of God and Poet." This verse is closely linked to what I have called the *creational* process, ever since I started working on the interlocution between the work of Freud, Goethe and Vicente Huidobro's creationism and vision of the poet as a "little god", in the previous chapters. Shelley's proposal is allied to this attempt to elucidate the workings of the immense internal universe that lives in each of us.

Notes

1 Drummond, perhaps, would have preferred that this theorisation be in verse: "the ambiguous cloud that is diluted in this object that is vaguer than a cloud and more defenceless – the body! Body, body, / truth so final, thirst so varied, / and that horse loose in the bed, / walking across the chest of the one who loves." Excerpt from the poem "*O quarto em desordem*", in *Fazendeiro do ar* (Drummond, (1954) 2014).

2 Communicating with all the analysand's internal psychic regions is in line with the thinking of Danielle Quinodoz and Christopher Bollas. See Part I, Chapter 14, "Other authors and different approaches to psychoanalytic work from the couch", and Part I, Chapter 7, "Christopher Bollas and the evocative couch".

3 For more on the cleavages in Freud's work, see Lora, Paim Filho and Nunes, 2018.

4 For a discussion of the terms, see Drawin and Moreira, 2018.

5 Freud, (1918 [1914]) 2010b.

6 Freud, (1911) 2010a, pp. 13–107.

7 Freud, (1896) 1996b.

8 Freud uses the term hallucinatory paranoia when referring to this case on p. 596 of *The Interpretation of Dreams* [(1900) 2019].

9 According to James Strachey's commentary, this would be the first time that Freud used the term projection in a publication: "In paranoia, self-accusation is repressed by a process that can be described as *projection*." [Freud, (1896) 1996b, p. 182.]

10 Freud, (1905 [1901]) 2016.

11 See Part I, Chapter 7, "Christopher Bollas and the evocative couch".

12 Bollas, 2000a.

13 However, Bollas works from his theories, using different nomenclature to the one I have chosen to use here, in order to make it easier for the Freudian reader to understand.

14 Freud, (1950 [1895]) 1996; Freud, (1905) 2016a.

15 Freud, (1900) 2019, p. 122.

16 "Moreover, let us recall that this transformation of representations into sensory images does not occur only in dreams, but also in hallucinations, in visions that may appear independently under conditions of health, or as symptoms of the psychoneuroses." [Freud, (1900) 2019, p. 586.]

17 We could think of two main ways of accessing the primitive. One would be to access something of the order of primitive content; the other would be to access and "work" from a more primitive mode of functioning. Artistic creation, for example, would be one of the ways of accessing a primitive mode functioning – accessing the *creational*, which creates the world and itself.

18 Freud, (1900) 2019, p. 595.

19 When theorising about dreams and the symptoms (theorising that also helps us to think about transference and session work), Freud tells us about the three facets of regression: "a) a topological regression, in the sense of the schema of the systems; b) a temporal one, when it is a return to older psychic formations; and c) a formal regression, when primitive modes of expression and representation replace the usual ones." [Freud, (1900) 2019, p. 599.]

20 Abraham, (1924) 1970.

21 As seen in the clinical examples of Winnicott, Ogden and many others, in Part I, Chapter 14, "Other authors and different approaches to psychoanalytic work from the couch".

22 However, they are "felt" by the analyst through his *reverie* and countertransference.

23 The clinical examples reported by the authors in this book can be correlated with my propositions.

24 Furthermore, this form of object relationship would only be displaced into the analysis (in order to be worked through), since it would already be operating, in a way, in the analysand's object relationships in their life beyond the sessions.

25 Even though the analyst's faults can be very productive for the analysis process, if he or she is able to recognise them in front of the analysand.

26 See Chapter 4, "Didier Anzieu's skin couch".

27 This idea of cell death and renewal as a metaphor for thinking about psychism was introduced by Sabina Spielrein [(1912) 2021, pp. 20–21].

28 In some cases, only when they requested it; in others, it was already made available beforehand, every time they entered the reception room.

29 Two sessions a week, lying on the couch.

30 Also neurotic regions, which led her to lead a minimally functional life, within her means and despite the intense suffering.

31 "Lubricating" speech should be seen from a broad perspective, and can be understood as "libidinising" speech, "sexualising" speech, if we are thinking from the point of view of Freudian metapsychology. As well as meeting physiological needs, water in a session can also be understood in a metaphorical way, as covering up or symbolically replacing "something". In this analysand's case, water could be seen as a symbolic substitute for breast milk.

32 In no way do I intend to generalise the analysand's way of dressing as being linked to some kind of psychic suffering. My comments refer exclusively to the case in question and only to its singularity.

33 The material from her treatment leads me to understand that her husband suffered from a more severe psychic condition than she did. He would not go out into the street, spent money he did not have (taking it from her), was an absent father, and, as her analysis progressed, he seemed increasingly encapsulated and isolated within the home, without any productive activity, while his eating compulsion grew, having already led him to a considerable state of morbid obesity.

34 See the autistic-contiguous position in Part I, Chapter 6, "Thomas Ogden and privacy on the couch".

35 A womb-couch, gestational of becoming, of *re-forming*.

36 As well as its metabolic-psychic capacity. We could think about this metabolic-psychic capacity, for example, based on the contributions of Ernst Simmel and Jean

Laplanche. The former presents us with a psychic model inspired by a digestive model, in which the psyche functions in a gastrointestinal way. The latter, in turn, presents a translation model, in which a psyche is always internally translating (and metabolising) what comes from the psyche of another [Simmel, (1943), 2022; Laplanche, 1985].

37 I repeat: I'm only talking about my clinic here. At least, there hasn't been a case that has made me rethink this position.

38 Or kind of "corporeal" receptacle, performing a *containerised* function of their own psyche.

39 It's at the service of abstinence.

40 See Part I, Chapter 9, "René Roussillon's couch in latency".

41 This example should not be understood in a concrete way. The content of your enunciation should be more specific and not as extensive as in the example. It's also important to remember what has been worked on in each individual assessment process. Otherwise, our protective care, when it comes to pointing out the couch, would end up being an excess, which would make it difficult for the analysand to metabolise.

42 I'll explain below why I say something similar to that.

43 A single statement by the analyst can be essentially paradoxical, containing at the same time what refers to playfulness and what belongs to the order of a limit (boundary, law, castration, etc.), depending on the context.

44 Aline Bei poetically writes: "I'd like to know how the body feels living like this, in the cloud" (2017).

45 See Part I, Chapter 7, "Christopher Bollas and the evocative couch".

46 See again Part I, Chapter 1, "Sigmund Freud's couch-reminiscence".

47 See again Part I, Chapter 9, "René Roussillon's couch in latency".

48 Freud, (1912–1913) 2012.

49 This aesthetic choice certainly ends up influencing and "permeating" the free association of my analysands, since the movement of the clouds and their forms are often explicitly communicated by the analysands throughout their process.

50 See again Part I, Chapter 7, "Christopher Bollas and the evocative couch".

51 Bringing things from home and/or something that symbolises the session is a recurring theme in children's clinics.

52 As an aside for the reader of this English edition: the rivalry between the football clubs of Porto Alegre (Internacional and Grêmio) is considered the greatest in Brazil, and even in Latin America. Supporting one of these teams is part of the local culture, with roughly half of the city (and indeed the state) supporting each club.

53 See the chapter "Some considerations on the history and etymology of the word couch".

54 As for thinking about objects of use in childcare, I have previously discussed the use of musical instruments in the text "Clinical sonorities" (Krüger, 2017a).

55 See Part I, Chapter 10, "The analyst's creative process and the couch for Melanie Klein".

56 Part I, Chapter 14, "Other authors and different approaches to psychoanalytic work from the couch" compiles some of this material.

57 Ferenczi, (1931) 2011b, pp. 69–83.

58 Milner, (1948) 1991, pp. 74–79. *Note*: This idea of the adult analysand requesting extra auxiliary objects is interesting, and perhaps we should discuss it further on another occasion.

59 Excerpt from "Segundo dia 2.2", a poem from *Livro das ignorãças* (Barros, (1993), 2013.

60 Freud, (1900) 2019.

61 Among other passages, we can find this use of *Übertragung* in Freud, (1900) 2019, p. 614.
62 Freud, (1895) 1996a.
63 See Part II, Chapter 20, "The cloud, condensation and poetic creation: reflections on the *Dichter*, *Dichtung* and *Verdichtung*".
64 Freud, (1900) 2019, p. 586.
65 Excerpt from the poem "Jet-lagged", by Waly Salomão, in the book *Algaravias: Câmara de ecos* [(1996) 2014].
66 Shelley, (1840 [1815]) 2008, pp. 117–118.

Final words

The reader has certainly realised that the second part of this book contains ideas that go beyond a mere reflecting on the status of the couch in psychoanalysis. It would not be possible for me to share my current view on the subject without evoking all this theoretical-clinical thinking and the way I have been listening to and carrying out my psychoanalytic work at the moment.

I believe it is essential that the entire psychoanalytic community and its members can share their concerns with their colleagues. I may well continue to work on the proposals in this book, which go beyond thinking about the couch, in new publications. It is also possible that I will reformulate them or even abandon them, as Freud did throughout his work. The internal movement never stops. For me, it is indisputable that one of the fundamental values of psychoanalytic theoretical-clinical work is that psychoanalysts circulate their unique thinking among their peers, regardless of the effects and types of repercussions they may cause in the subsequent exchange between colleagues.

My vision of the clinic has become increasingly inseparable from artistic and poetic endeavours. With this in mind, I have tried to develop this proposal as thoroughly as the moment allows, knowing that each parallel theme could well be elaborated differently in specific works dedicated to it.

From the first part of the book, the reader will have noticed my impetus to justify the importance of using the couch-object in analysis, and I hope I have made it clear that I am not referring to the importance of its use only in what is conventionally called classical psychoanalysis. Even when we work with analysands in whom non-neurotic regions predominate, I don't think we should change the nomenclature of our work to "psychotherapy" or any other term. Since Freud, psychoanalysis has been psychotherapy in itself. Where there is a psychoanalyst carefully working through all the technical intricacies, and an analysand who desires the process, regardless of the order of their suffering, we are always talking about an analysis.

DOI: 10.4324/9781003681212-26

From the beginning I approached the question of the use or non-use of the couch by way of other authors, in order to make it very clear that highlighting the importance of its use is not a conservative position; on the contrary. Contemporary tendencies to relativise the use of the couch based on prerogatives that do not seem to me any deeper than those presented here led me to write this book. **It is necessary that we re-listen, re-read, re-interpret and, above all, *re-form* the function of the couch in the psychoanalytic clinic.**

The book project didn't include a discussion of remote *online* work,[1] which is due to the fact that I do not regard it as antagonistic to working on the *couch/diwan*, as I have developed in Part II. In a certain sense, the remote and online question concerns more what is linked to the conditions of the setting, from an external point of view. Everything that has been clinically considered from the broad notion of the *couch/diwan* would encompass online treatment and has its analogues within this modality of setting. I believe that the online modality should operate as an adjustment to what is possible, within its limitations, of all that has been proposed regarding the *couch/diwan*, the work from the cloud state and all the propositions already discussed, transferring the critique related to face-to-face to that of screen-to-screen.

It seems to me that we should take Ferenczi's elasticity of technique in this sense: as an elasticity of technique, of listening, of interventions, of the very modality of conceiving the session – not necessarily a matter of rethinking the use of the couch as a device, even if we may endlessly *re-form* the way we approach it.

It would be naïve and simplistic to imagine that the problems and difficulties of technique with difficult analysands are located in the use of the couch, or to follow an unfortunate statement by Elisabeth Roudinesco when she claims: "Psychoanalysis must evolve at the pace imposed by the world. It should focus on shorter treatments, during which the patient is interacted with face to face, and not on the couch."[2] Now, the rhythm of an analysis is never that imposed by the world; at most, it is the rhythm dictated by the internal. To follow such a proposition without reflecting on the depth of the work that the couch offers us, from what has been seen through all the authors mentioned, and what we have subsequently developed with regard to the metaphor of the cloud, is sad and reductionist for psychoanalysis, not to say more.

Carrying out an analysis at the pace imposed by the world or by the conscious desire of the analysand (when they say they "prefer" to be analysed face-to-face), without taking into account all the complex discussions set out in this book, is almost as if we analysts were saying: "Let's work on fortifying a *false self* and move on." The seriousness of Roudinesco's statement is even greater, as it is made in the *newspaper El País*, which means expanding her position outside the psychoanalytic sphere; and still worse: without raising the discussion to its appropriate level of complexity.[3] Her position, at no point, rests on the clinic, but rather reduces the analytic session to a formality in order to comply with the demands of the external world, without any concern for discussing the functionality of the couch. I repeat, it's not a question of denying a possible eye-to-eye treatment, but the criterion certainly couldn't be on account of a manifest desire on the part of the analysand; there would have to be much deeper justifications than that, as discussed throughout this book. There are fellow psychoanalysts who find them in their own way, based on their clinical practice and their listening, and I owe them the greatest respect. However, as has been explained so far, working on the analytic process using the *couch/diwan* has been fundamental in the processes of analysis that I conduct, regardless of the "psychopathological types" present in my clinic.[4] My intention is that what has been problematised in this writing may mobilise the discussion around the false dichotomy: couch = classical analysis (neuroses), face-to-face = non-neuroses.

I believe that if the handling is "good enough", taking into account tact, holding, and the various propositions offered throughout this book, there would be no reason to consider the couch, concretely, as a problem *a priori* for the treatment of so-called "difficult cases". A*s our popular saying goes, "the matter runs deeper than that"*. It seems to me that the proposition of face-to-face treatments has become increasingly trivialised today, often much more due to analysts' difficulties in managing the couch beyond classical listening and intervention than because the couch itself would be an impediment. Of course, we cannot treat the couch as an untouchable god, which could never be abandoned, but, on the other hand, neither can we categorically state that it could not be of use in such cases.[5]

As developed throughout this book, the point lies elsewhere; hence we must ask whether, at times, the analyst may not be "resisting" the use of the couch in certain clinical circumstances, as a form of secondary gain (that is, avoiding aspects of the analysand's primitive functioning which could only emerge through this medium – a "harder" work, which would unsettle the analyst more). However, I repeat, I don't intend to be dogmatic and I believe that we should always re-evaluate whether or not, for whatever reason, a case should be treated off the couch. However, I simply believe that face-to-face should not be seen as the "new normal" or that the use of the couch is obsolete, as Roudinesco seemed to signal.

Certainly, this book's discussions also cover group sessions and/or situations where there is no basic infrastructure for working with the couch – such as sessions aimed at low-income populations in places where it is not possible to create an environment with the comfort of a consulting room. The question of comfort is indeed an important one to raise, because, without a doubt, the comfort of both analyst and analysand supports the analytic process. In all areas of life, especially outside the psychoanalytic context, comfort aids the fullest development of whatever is at stake. Hunger reduces the very possibility of complexifying any process – and, consequently, the psychoanalytic process itself. "As if the city did not serve us its bread of clouds," says Drummond's poem.[6]

In this sense, we can't be hypocrites. I must emphasise that I'm talking about optimal conditions for conducting an analysis – which is not always possible – but this does not prevent the questions raised here from reverberating in some way within other modalities of psychoanalytic practice.

The purpose of this work is to re-think and *re-form* the status of the couch for when there is the material possibility of working from it. Psychoanalytic work is always a work of hope, a work aimed at changing the world – whether internal or external. It is up to us, psychoanalysts, to make use as profoundly as possible of the resources at our disposal. If not the couch, then at least the cloud is offered – in one way or another – to all.

Ra[7]
I have the morning
glowing) strong inside the eye

The embryo of the embrace
crossing the eyelid of the skyscraper

I have the cloud
playing around my fingers
transforming what lives within reality[8]

Notes

1 One extended version of "The need for the couch or a substitute other than the gaze" was included in this book as an extra text, in order to address this issue in some way (Kupermann, Gondar and Dal Molin, 2022).
2 Interview with Élisabeth Roudinesco (2015). Available at: brasil.elpais.com/brasil/2015/09/02/cultura/1441210297_491115.html.
3 I confess that I like the idea of believing that Roudinesco's statement is a misinterpretation on the part of her interviewer and that she didn't actually say what was published in this way.
4 Only what I experience from it can I share with my colleagues. Confrontations about this are welcome, and there is a considerable bibliography that confronts it throughout the book.
5 A discourse that we often see replicated.
6 Excerpt from the poem "Hotel Toffolo" [Drummond de Andrade, (1951a) 2014, p. 345]. In the same book, Drummond also leaves us verses that help us think about working with sadness, evoking the figure of the cloud: "[…] And it remains, / lost in the air, why better to keep it, / a particular sadness, stamping its seal on the clouds" ("Tarde de Mayo", Drummond de Andrade, (1951b) 2014, pp. 326–327).
7 Sun God of Ancient Egypt.
8 Poem from the book *Homenagem à nuvem* (Krüger, 2017b, p. 88).

Extras

Creation poem

Through this QR code, the poem printed in black-and-white on the right-hand page can be visualised with a blue background and words written in white, respecting the author's aesthetic intention (and relating more deeply to his metaphor about the cloud state).

DOI: 10.4324/9781003681212-28

pá
larva

ímã
gene

nada

palavra

imagem

nada

palavra imaginada

Poem Criação (Creation) by Lucas Krüger, in the book Homenagem à nuvem (Homage to the Cloud), 2017.

Note on untranslatability

This visual poem remains in Portuguese. Its structure relies on the internal play of the Portuguese language: the splitting and recombination of words such as *pá* (spade), *larva* (larva), *imã* (magnet), *gene* (gene), and *nada* (nothing), which, when read in sequence, reverberate into *palavra* (word), *imagem* (image), and *palavra imaginada* (imagined word).

The semantic and phonetic condensations here are inseparable from Portuguese morphology and sound.

Any literal translation would flatten this complexity, reducing what is essentially a poetic experiment in the materiality of language – its echoes, gaps and metamorphoses – into a mere set of dictionary correspondences. What is at stake is not only the meaning of the words, but their very ability to transform into one another, to conceal and reveal simultaneously.

For this reason, the poem is preserved in its original language, allowing the English-speaking reader to encounter the opacity and strangeness of Portuguese itself – much as a psychoanalytic session encounters the foreignness of the unconscious.

Provocative considerations on remote online sessions

The need for the couch or a substitute other than the gaze

Editorial note: This is a version of the text originally published in the book *Ferenczi: Thinker of Catastrophe*, organised by Daniel Kupermann, Jô Gondar and Eugênio Canesin Dal Molin (2022). The book was organised in such a way that the text by one author (Bruna Zerbinatti) is presented as a provocation-stimulus for the text by a second author (Renato Mezan) and, even later, by a third author (in this case, me, Lucas Krüger). The version published here is the one presented at an event at the Sigmund Freud Psychoanalytic Association (Porto Alegre) on 5 October 2022, with minor changes. It's also important to point out that this text was published during the writing of this book. I could say that its content is largely a summary of what is proposed more closely in the chapters on Ferenczi, Winnicott and Green, although some reflections are found exclusively here.[1]

*

I will follow the organisers' request to add a "third layer" to the elements that colleagues Bruna Paola Zerbinatti and Renato Mezan have brought into the discussion. I will not comment directly on the content of their writings, though I accompany them in a latent way.

Zerbinatti evokes the notions of rhythm and tempo while Mezan follows the music in order to explain the measures didactically, working on the notions of silence, space and the body, and both culminate, each in their own way, in a discussion about psychoanalytic listening and the challenges of *online* clinical work. I intend to follow their writing project, which, in a nutshell, will move from a musical reflection to a reflection on the body and presence and will end with the question of the couch, to finally problematise remote online treatment. The reader will realise that Mezan's quote from Otto Fenichel, "When one cannot be 'classical', a 'non-classical' procedure is equally psychoanalytic", will be an important trigger for our discussion.

Sándor Ferenczi is the first psychoanalyst to be effectively concerned with musical language. In his text *The Interpretation of the Melodies that Come into Our Minds* (1909)[2] – although only published posthumously – we can perceive Ferenczi's tact[3] towards the theme musicality and "sound associations not

DOI: 10.4324/9781003681212-29

determined by the content of words". Freud[4] was more familiar with the subject, referring to the "sound image" as the link between the representation of a word and the representation of a thing. "But yes, there are melodies without words (melodies without text that come to mind, like symphonies, sonatas, etc.)," says Ferenczi,[5] who wonders if rhythm is a correspondent of humour. "The degree of my joy, or even my sadness, corresponds exactly to the rhythm of the melody that comes to mind," he observes.

By considering that he was not a musician, Ferenczi suggests that a musician with psychoanalytic training could better develop what he shares without further elaboration in this writing, which may have been the reason why it was only published posthumously. However, we note that the theme of melody runs through his clinical practice, and we can see it in *Prolongations of the 'Active Technique' in Psychoanalysis* (1921), a text in which Ferenczi presents a clinical section in which a particular melody is a trigger for working on an analysand's psychic contents. In the case in question, the melody, the singing and the piano playing in session would have helped to unveil aspects of the analysand's sexuality and childhood conflicts, closely linked to her body and her bodily activity – which involved controlling her anal and urethral sphincters, as well as clitoral masturbation. We're not interested in discussing Ferenczi's active technique here, nor should we go into more detail on the case. It seems interesting to think about what is implied: the musical instrument used as a bodily extension. In describing how man has built civilisation and his tools, Freud states that "through each instrument, man recreates his own organs, motor or sensory, or extends the limits of their functioning".[6] Although Freud is not referring specifically to the musical instrument, his claim certainly encompasses it.[7] We may then ask: Could we not think of the couch, an instrument (in the broad sense) of the psychoanalyst, from the corporeal perspective to which Freud alludes?

Today we know,[8] due to advances in medicine, that the tactile and auditory senses are prominent in the life of the foetus, and that it even dreams of "sound images". The rhythm of the mother's and foetus' heartbeats, as well as the blood flow, are present from the tactile bodily vibration of intrauterine life and become more complex as the auditory system develops. Winnicott probably already sensed the importance of this primordial tactile-auditory experience, and opened up the possibility of thinking of the use of the couch (and listening from it) as a supporting instrument-object, an instrument that can complement and/or extend the body, just as in the mother-baby relationship, as we can see in the following passages.

> The couch and cushions are there for the patient to use. They will appear in thoughts and dreams, in which case they will represent the analyst's body, their breasts, arms, hands, etc., in an infinite variety of forms. To the extent that the patient is regressed (for a moment or an hour, or for a long period of time), the couch is the analyst, the pillows *are* breasts, the analyst *is* the

> mother at a certain time in the past. In extreme situations, the couch can no longer be said to represent the analyst.
>
> For the neurotic, the couch, warmth and comfort can *symbolise* the mother's love. For the psychotic, it would be more accurate to say that these things *are* the physical expression of the analyst's love. The couch *is* the analyst's lap or womb, and the warmth *is* the warmth of the analyst's body. And so on and so forth.[9]

Note that Winnicott is also thinking of using the couch with "severe cases", explicitly citing psychosis. We know that Winnicott[10] emphasises the need for the creative omnipotence of the baby, present in the *moment of* initial *illusion of* the mother-baby relationship, for the processes of integration (or non-integration of the *self*). The psychoanalyst Margaret Little, who called herself a *psycho-borderline*, reports that, in her analysis (on the couch) with Winnicott, she was in moments of extreme regression, completely covered by a blanket, and also holding hands with Winnicott. "DW didn't represent my mother to me. In my illusion of transference, he was my mother. As there is in fact continuity between mother and foetus, genetic and physical, for me his hands were the umbilical cord, his couch the placenta and the blanket the membranes ..."[11]

> Literally, for endless hours, he held my two hands tightly between his, almost like an umbilical cord, while I lay there, often hidden under the blanket, silent, inert, withdrawn, terrified, angry or in tears, asleep and sometimes dreaming.[12]

The excerpts from Winnicott highlighted above, together with Little's accounts, as well as the case described in the text *Withdrawal and Regression*,[13] reinforce the use of the couch as an instrument-object of auxiliary use for analysis in any type of psychic illness. From this point of view, the couch is there to be used in whatever way the analysand needs, symbolically or not, bodily or not, neurotically or not. We can also add that the couch fulfils the function of a third object. Winnicott[14] explains that the regression to dependence (brought about by the use of the couch) is "an integral part of analysing the phenomena of early childhood, and if the couch gets wet, the patient gets dirty or drools, we will know that these things are inherent and not a complication". Ferenczi would likely have been enthusiastic about Winnicott's comments that we are quoting, and could add that "... we even let the patient immerse himself in all the early stages of passive object love, where, in murmured phrases, like a child about to fall asleep, he allows us to glimpse his oneiric universe".[15] But why am I writing about the couch-instrument, if our proposal is to reflect on online remote treatment? Well, both Renato Mezan and Bruna Paola Zerbinatti mentioned, *en passant* (because it's not the main object of their reflections), a dichotomy between treatments using the couch versus face-to-face ones – and

I believe this issue deserves to be deepened before we turn to the online modality.

It is noteworthy that a strong current of thought among contemporary psychoanalysts holds that "severe cases" must be treated face-to-face, grounding their positions essentially on the necessity of the gaze. By no means do I intend to dismantle such positions – which are and must be thought from within the clinic – but rather to continue problematising the issue. Even though Ferenczi[16] sometimes affirmed that he would allow the analysand to forgo the couch in order to say something while looking him in the eye, and even though we have other reports of clinical situations outside the couch – such as the piano playing and role-plays combined with play ("analysis through play", by Ferenczi),[17] it would not be true to say that Ferenczi sought to contemplate an indication of face-to-face to the detriment of the couch. I understand that his "elastic technique" is much more related to the idea of facilitating the emergence of the child who lives in the adult than any reflection on the importance of the concrete gaze (because the analysand "looks" when listening, and the analysand is "looked at" when listened to), although it would also not be true to say that Ferenczi was opposed to face-to-face consultations, not least because his work is characterised by experimentation. However, I understand that the essence of his thinking, as well as Winnicott's, is to emphasise the importance of play as an aid to the analysis of adults, and this would not necessarily involve a proposal to defend a face-to-face modality (which we take here as analogous to the use of the screen in online treatment).

In *Aims of Psychoanalytic Treatment*,[18] Winnicott reports practising *modified analysis*, though without specifying exactly what this meant, stating only that he usually tried to adhere as closely as possible to a standard analysis, yet without hesitation in "practising something else"[19] – and without alluding to the necessity of the gaze and/or the face-to-face modality.

We find theoretical elaborations and clinical cases from psychoanalysts such as Christopher Bollas, Thomas Ogden, James Grotstein, Didier Anzieu, Masud Khan, among others, who each in their own way highlight a bodily function allied to the primary object of care – in a manner similar to what we pointed out through Winnicott – with the caveat, perhaps, that Margaret Little's treatment is the only one in which we find an account where the analyst's body, beyond the couch, ends up being materially used.

As for emphasising the importance of the couch even in more severe cases, my position is not to uphold a conservative or dogmatic attitude towards the couch, but to problematise the issue. As didactically written by Renato Mezan, André Green gives us a real lesson on the frame, especially about the importance of the internal frame, but I'll be bold enough to point out some passages by Green – not the ones selected by Mezan – about the need for the gaze in session that are confusing, to say the least.

In an interview with Fernando Urribarri, Green defends the idea of the "good enough mother" as the founder of the framing structure:

> What do *hold* and *handle* mean for the baby being held? What does it mean? Well, precisely: a framing structure. When you're separated from your mother, it's not the memory of her face or her smile that matters. What counts are the traces of the frame that the contact of her body represented. Mother's face and smile can disappear or be replaced. The frame remains.[20]

Green quotes Winnicott to emphasise that the frame provided by being in the mother's arms, lap and body is more important than the distinctive configuration of her features and eye contact with her. However, in the same interview, he says that, in severe cases, it is necessary to modify the frame and come to accept face-to-face treatment because of the gaze.[21] Now, if Green affirms that the framing of the body in the mother's arms is more important than the gaze, why does his clinical justification for the face-to-face setting rely primarily on the gaze?

This is contradictory, because in the interview with Urribarri, in order to articulate the idea of face-to-face sessions over against the couch, Green cites Winnicott's text *Hate in the Counter-Transference* (1947)[22] and, to defend the same point, in his book *Guidelines for a Contemporary Psychoanalysis*,[23] Green also cites Winnicott – this time, the text *Clinical and Metapsychological Aspects of Regression in the Psychoanalytic Context* ([1954a] 1993),[24] which, of course, is an even greater incongruity, since not only does Winnicott make no mention in favour of switching from the couch to face-to-face, but even in both of the texts cited by Green, Winnicott emphasises the couch as a possible "mother's body" and the possibility of analysis unfolding from that very understanding. Therefore, in order to defend the face-to-face and the need for the gaze in non-neurotic cases, Green essentially used the texts in which Winnicott demonstrates an interesting use of the couch in non-neurotic cases.

It is through a contradictory reading of Winnicott's writings that Green articulates the face-to-face and the importance of the gaze in the *setting*. The question that remains is: If Green himself says that the mother's body/setting is more important than the gaze, why would he defend the gaze, giving up the couch (based on Winnicott, precisely in the texts in which he proposes that we think of the couch as the mother's body, and which even try to work on a deep regression to dependence that takes place on the couch)?[25]

Green's misreading does not diminish the importance of his thought, nor does it diminish the problematisation of the gaze as a possible aid to treatment. If Green were faithful to his own assertion that the frame/mother's body is more important than the gaze, and if he wished to rely on Winnicott to defend a practice, it seems to me that Green should have stated that, rather than the gaze, the analysand – even one with a severe pathology – ought to lie on the couch, since that frame would refer back to the mother's body (the structuring frame) and the couch to the function of holding and handling, which are more fundamental than the gaze (according to Green's own statement). Or else, in order to emphasise the importance of the concreteness of the gaze, Green would have had to seek another conceptual basis to defend the face-to-face setting, rather than the very sources he chose to draw upon in Winnicott's work. For it is implicit in Winnicott's thought that the way the analyst handles and holds the analysand within the frame is what truly matters. Such a theoretical-clinical contradiction simply makes clear to us how complex and diverse the positions can be regarding the possible uses – and non-uses – of the couch.

Respecting the positions that defend the importance of the face-to-face setting, my clinical experience leads me to stress the importance of the use of the couch-instrument even in "difficult cases", in which issues related to what we could understand as "non-integration" or "disintegration" prevail. It is through the couch that I conduct these "modified analyses" – to use Winnicott's term, in contrast to "classical analysis". And it is from my experience that I came to reflect on Bruna Paola Zerbinatti's proposal concerning intervals of speech/silence and tempo. I understand that "modified analysis", whether in-person or remote, requires more "modifications" of the classical technique than the replacement of the couch (or some substitute, such as the analysand's bed, in the case of remote analysis) by the face-to-face mode. What seems more pressing is to take into greater account holding, handling and the broadening of ways of listening and intervening on the couch, rather than to abdicate the potentiality of this instrument.

"Analysis through play" presupposes that the analyst "participates" more actively through their speech and mental constructions than in a "classic analysis". So, taking my colleagues' (Mezan and Zerbinatti's) theorising about silences and progress, I'm inclined to think that "difficult cases" demand a greater "continuity of voice" (as a presence) from the analyst, whether the sessions are face-to-face or online.[26]

As I work essentially with the use of the couch (we're talking about adult analysands), I have to confess that I didn't feel any greater fatigue (compared to what is essential) in carrying out predominantly online consultations, as Zerbinatti problematised. My consultations were carried out without looking directly at each other, so this point wasn't so difficult – though singular – in most cases. The difficulty that affected some treatments, especially the more "difficult" ones, was precisely the interval – felt as a rupture – of the use of the couch as a bodily continuity and/or as a support in the sense of the "mother's body", a feeling of loss of the object of use that had an important sustaining function. These analysands did not claim to miss the in-person sessions and/or my "physical presence", but, already in the first online sessions, they expressed missing, literally, the couch and even its cushion. In fact, the couch had fulfilled a supportive function, and as cosy as it might have seemed to use their "own" bed,[27] in their "own" home, as a substitute for the function the couch had once fulfilled, the "loss" of it was traumatic and disorganizing – and each case had to be handled singularly. We are speaking of cases in which it is anything but simple to live "well enough" with oneself.

It is of course clear that colleagues may object to the defence of the couch in such cases. Undoubtedly, we are not speaking of an "easy" analytic process. Nevertheless, I believe it is necessary to emphasise that the concreteness of the gaze seems to me to hinder rather than help the necessary regression/regredience to the primitive periods (or psychic locations) where the "greyish" nuclei of the traumatic and/or psychotic parts of the self generally reside. We know that such issues involve excessive experiences. On this point, Thomas Ogden (2013) can contribute to the discussion by highlighting the analysand's need (and also the analyst's) for privacy in the use of the couch, where there is a space that belongs only to the analysand, a space that belongs only to the analyst, and a third intersubjective space that is shared (the analytic third). For him, the privacy afforded by working on the couch is essential for both analysand and analyst to surrender themselves fully to free association and evenly suspended attention. Therefore, not being face-to-face with the analysand is also essential for the analyst to achieve the "immersion" that psychoanalytic listening demands. Let us not forget that we too need to be in good condition to listen deeply.[28] We "look" at our analysands when we truly listen to them.

We can't deny that working with images is fundamental to the analytical process, but the work becomes more profound if these are "mental images" offered by the psychoanalyst, rather than the analyst's actual image. As Mezan pointed out, the voice is a corporeal representative of the analyst, and it still seems to me to be our richest tool for intervention, especially if it is aided by the framing corporeal aspects of the couch (or a substitute that fulfils its function, in the case of online work).

It's important not to confuse the concrete gaze with acceptance, or to accuse the couch of providing distance (or even coldness). Let's not project this onto it and let's reflect on the issue of welcoming, encompassing the multiple functions of the couch. It's good to remember that the concrete gaze is not and never has been "forbidden" in a treatment that prioritises the couch, because by simply turning their head, the analysand will see the analyst and make sure they are physically present when necessary.

The point is that working on the couch with difficult cases demands more from the analyst. It requires the analyst to have undergone a profound personal analysis, to possess a high capacity for holding and handling, and, above all, to withstand the emergence of the traumatic core. To work in this way is to make oneself available to work at the deepest level of Ferenczi's empathy (*Einfühlung*), welcoming (or recovering) the child who lives in the adult. To offer mental images, rather than facilitating a narcissistic capture by the self-image, is to offer the capacity to play and the capacity for creative omnipotence, so that the analysand may create/re-create/transform/*re-form* their sick inner world into one in which life predominates.

In this short piece of writing, I've made a great effort to try to convey these reflections in the most thorough way possible. However, I'm afraid I've left too many gaps that could be better explored and discussed, so I hope that this can be done at a later date, and I also hope that this "third layer" of reflection contributes to the complexity of what Zerbinatti and Mezan have brought. The questions I would like to leave reverberating are: Should the couch not be seen more as an ally than as an obstacle in severe pathologies? Should we not pay greater attention to the paradox that inhabits the couch (or its analogous substitute), rather than viewing it solely through the lens of "classical analysis," as representing lack, absence (which, in difficult cases, would leave the analysand in the void), and re-think it also as a body-object-instrument that aids the necessary holding in such treatments? And finally: How can we continue problematizing these questions in the context of remote online treatments?

Notes

1 Krüger, 2022.
2 This title refers to the translation of the text made from the German by E. Spieler, F. Gerchman and myself for the book *Dreams, Melodies and Symptoms*, a selection of texts by Ferenczi. The original title of the text is *Zur Deutung einfallander Melodien*. See Ferenczi, (1909) 2019.
3 Ferenczi, (1909) 2019, p. 14.
4 Freud, (1915), 1996, pp. 217–222.
5 Ferenczi, 1909, p. 14.
6 Freud, (1930) 2006a, p. 97.
7 In *Clinical Sonorities*, I tried to elucidate, through various clinical situations, some of the specific functions that particular musical instruments can fulfil in analyses with children, especially with regard to issues related to the body.
8 Maíra dos Santos Jaber works on my statement (summarised here) in much more detail in her dissertation (2013).
9 Winnicott, (1954a) 2000a, pp. 285, 283.
10 Winnicott, (1945a) 1982; Winnicott, (1945b) 1982.
11 Little, (1990) 1992, pp. 95–96.
12 Little, (1990) 1992, p. 46.
13 Winnicott, (1954a) 2000a.
14 Winnicott, (1954b) 2000a, p. 386.
15 Winnicott, (1954a) 2000a, p. 386.
16 Ferenczi, (1930) 1992a, p. 58.
17 Ferenczi, (1931) 2011b, p. 69.
18 Winnicott, (1962) 1984.
19 Both the terms in inverted commas and those in italics come from Winnicott himself.
20 Green and Urribarri, 2019, pp. 64–65.
21 Green and Urribarri, 2019, p. 70.
22 Winnicott, (1947) 2000.
23 Green, 2008, p. 49.
24 Precisely the texts from which we have taken the excerpts quoted above.
25 However, despite Green's theorising, as presented in Part I, Chapter 5, *André Green's couch – the dream model, other contributions and misreadings*, it is possible to find clinical reports by Green involving the treatment of "difficult cases" on the couch.
26 We could think of these statements, for example, in the light of René Roussillon's concept of "psychoanalytic conversation" (Roussillon, (2005) 2005/2).

27 I'm referring to the bed because it seems to me to be the ideal substitute for the couch in remote treatment, since it refers to the most intimate, to the bedroom, to one's dream life and also to sexuality, even though we know it's not always possible to work in optimal conditions. It would be interesting to think of the bed and the bedroom from the perspective of what Christopher Bollas [(1989) 1992] calls evocative objectives.

28 Previously, Freud [(1913a) 1996e] had already pointed to the gaze as a hindrance to the listening process.

References

Abraham, Karl. *Selected Papers of Karl Abraham*. London: The International Psycho-Analytical Library; Hogarth Press and the Institute of PsychoAnalysis, 1942.

Abraham, Karl. Hysterical dream-states. *In*: Abraham, Karl. *Selected Papers of Karl Abraham*. London: The International Psycho-Analytical Library; Hogarth Press and the Institute of Psycho-Analysis, 1942a.

Abraham, Karl. Transformations of Scoptophilia. Hysterical dream-states. *In*: Abraham, Karl. *Selected Papers of Karl Abraham*. London: The International Psycho-Analytical Library; Hogarth Press and the Institute of Psycho-Analysis, 1942b.

Abraham, Karl (1909). *Sonho e mito: um estudo sobre a psicologia dos povos*. Translated by Lucas Krüger, Eduardo Spieler and Sander Machado da Silva. Porto Alegre: Artes & Ecos, 2020. (Série escrita psicanalítica.)

Abraham, K. (1924). A short study of the development of the libido. *In*: *Selected Papers of Karl Abraham*. London: The Hogarth Press, 1970.

Adler, G. (1988). How useful is the borderline concept? *Psychoanalytic Inquiry*, v. 8, n. 3, pp. 353–372

André, Jacques. Entrevista com Jacques André: a vida de hoje e a sexualidade de sempre. *Jornal de Psicanálise*, São Paulo, v. 42, n. 77, December 2009. Available at: pepsic.bvsalud.org/scielo.php?script=sci_arttext&pid=S0103-58352009000200002.

Anzieu, Didier. *O eu-pele*. Translated by Zakie Yazigi and Rosali Mahfuz. São Paulo: Casa do Psicólogo, 1989.

Anzieu, Didier. *A Skin for Thought: Interviews with Gilbert Tarrab on Psychology and Psychoanalysis*. London; New York: Karnac Books, 1990.

Bachelard, Gastón. As nuvens. *In*: *O ar e os sonhos*. Translated by Antônio Pádua Danesi. São Paulo: Martins Fontes, 1990.

Balint, Michael. *Thrills and Regressions*. New York: International Universities Press, 1959.

Baranger, Madeleine; Baranger, Willy (1961/1962). *La situación analítica como campo dinámico*. Problemas del campo psicoanalítico. Buenos Aires: Kargieman, 1969. Available at: https://www.apuruguay.org/apurevista/1960/16887247196119620401 01.pdf.

Barrento, João. As formas do informe. *In*: Goethe, Johann Wolfgang von. *O jogo das nuvens*. Selection, translation, preface and notes by João Barrento. Porto: Assírio & Alvim, 2003.

Barros, Manoel de (1993). Livro das ignorãças. *In*: Barros, Manoel de. *Poesia completa*. São Paulo: Leya, 2013.

Baudry, Francis. Greening of psychoanalysis: André Green's new paradigm in contemporary theory and practice. *Psychoanalytic Quarterly*, v. 87, n. 3, 2018.

Bei, Aline. *O peso do pássaro morto*. São Paulo: Editora Nós, 2017.

Bion, Wilfred R. (1957). Diferenciação entre a personalidade psicótica e a personalidade não-psicótica. *In*: Spillius, Elizabeth Bott. *Melanie Klein hoje: desenvolvimentos da teoria e da técnica*. Translated by B. H. Mandelbaum. Rio de Janeiro: Imago, 1991. v. 1.

Bion, Wilfred R. (1965). *Transformations*. London: Karnac, 1991a.

Bion, Wilfred R. (1975). *Clinical seminars and other works*. Karnac, 1994.

Bion, Wilfred R. (1978a). Brasília. *In*: Bion, Wilfred R. *Clinical Seminars and Other Works*. London: Karnac, 1994.

Bion, Wilfred R. *Cogitations*. London: Karnac, 2005.

Bion, Wilfred R. (1978b). *The Tavistock Seminars*. London; New York: Karnac, 2005.

Bion, Wilfred R. (1967). *Los Angeles Seminars and Supervision*. London: Karnac, 2013.

Bion, Wilfred R. (1978c). *Bion in New York and Sao Paulo and Three Tavistock Seminars*. London: The Harris Meltzer Trust, 2018.

Bion, Wilfred R. *Bion no Brasil: supervisões e comentários*. São Paulo: Blucher, 2018.

Bleger, José. Psicanálise do enquadramento psicanalítico. *In*: Bleger, José. *Simbiose e ambiguidade*. Translated by Maria Luiza de A. Borger. Rio de Janeiro: Francisco Alves, 1988.

Bollas, Christopher (1989). *Forças do destino*. São Paulo: Escuta, 1992.

Bollas, Christopher (1992). *Sendo um personagem*. Translated by Suzana Menescal de Alencar Carvalho. Technical review by José Outeiral. Rio de Janeiro: Revinter, 1998.

Bollas, Christopher. O estado de mente fascista. *In*: Bollas, Christopher. *Sendo um personagem*. Translated by S. M. A. Carvalho. Rio de Janeiro: Revinter, 1998.

Bollas, Christopher. *Hysteria*. São Paulo: Escuta, 2000a.

Bollas, Christopher (2000b). *Hysteria*. London; New York: Routledge, 2000a.

Bollas, Christopher. *The Freudian moment*. London: Karnac, 2007a.

Bollas, Christopher. *The evocative object world*. New York: Routledge, 2009.

Bollas, Christopher. Architecture and the unconscious. *In*: Bollas, Christopher. *The evocative object world*. New York: Routledge, 2009a.

Bollas, Christopher. *The infinite question*. London; New York: Routledge, 2009b.

Bollas, Christopher. *Catch them before they fall: the psychoanalysis of breakdown*. New York: Routledge, 2013.

Bollas, Christopher (2007b). *O momento freudiano*. São Paulo: Roca, 2013a.

Bollas, Christopher (1987a). *A sombra do objeto: psicanálise do conhecido não pensado*. Translated by Fátima Marques. São Paulo: Escuta, 2015.

Bollas, Christopher. *When the sun bursts: the enigma of schizophrenia*. New Haven: Yale University Press, 2015.

Bollas, Christopher (1987b). *The shadow of the object: psychoanalysis of the unthought known*. London; New York: Routledge, 2018a.

Bollas, Christopher. *Three characters: narcissist, borderline, manic depressive*. Bicester: Phoenix Publishing House, 2021.

Bolognini, Stefano. *Fluxos vitais: entre o self e o não self*. São Paulo: Blucher, 2022.

Botella, César; Botella, Sara. *The work of psychic figurability: mental states without representation*. East Sussex: Brunner-Routledge, 2005.

Bruni, Alessandro. Container-contained inverted relationship – (♀ ♂): developments and applications of a very powerful concept of Wilfred R. Bion. *In*: Levine, Howard B.; Brown, J. Lawrence (eds.). *Growth and turbulence in the container/contained: Bion's continuing legacy*. London: Routledge, 2013.

Busch, Fred. *Criar a mente psicanalítica*. Teoria e método psicanalítico. São Paulo: Escuta, 2017.

Campos, Haroldo de (1992). O que é mais importante: a escrita ou o escrito? Teoria da linguagem em Walter Benjamin. *In*: Tapia, Marcelo; Nóbrega, Thelma Médici (eds.). *Haroldo de Campos transcriação*. São Paulo: Perspectiva, 2015.

Cassorla, Roosevelt Moises S. (2013). Quando o analista se torna estúpido: tentativa de compreensão do enactment utilizando a teoria do pensamento de Bion. *In*: Barros Neto, Alberto Moniz da Rocha; Rocha, Elias Mallet da (eds.). *Psychoanalytic Quarterly – artigos contemporâneos de psicanálise*. São Paulo: Escuta, 2016. v. II.

Cassullo, Gabriele. The psychoanalytic contributions of Melitta Schmideberg Klein. More than Melanie Klein's rebel daughter. *The American Journal of Psychoanalysis*, v. 76, pp. 18–34, 2016.

Celenza, Andrea. Vis-à-vis the couch: Where is psychoanalysis? *International Journal of Psychoanalysis*, v. 86, pp. 1.645–1.659, 2005.

Civitarese, Giuseppe; Ferro, Antonino. *Playing and vitality in psychoanalysis*. Routledge, 2022.

Dejours, Christophe. O corpo inacabado entre fenomenologia e psicaná-lise: entrevista. *Dossiê: psicanálise e universidade São Paulo*, v. 26, n. 3, September–December, 2015. Available at: www.scielo.br/j/pusp/a/d766jpxNCfsX5rxqmr9yjxm/?lang=pt.

Deutsch, Felix. Analytic posturology. *Psychoanalytic Quarterly*, n. 21, pp. 196– 214, 1952.

Drawin, Carlos; Moreira, Jacqueline. A *Verleugnung* em Freud: análise textual e considerações hermenêuticas. *Psicologia USP, São Paulo*, v. 29, n. 1, January–April, 2018. Available at: https://doi.org/10.1590/0103-656420160171.

Drummond de Andrade, Carlos (1954). O quarto em desordem. *In*: Drummond de Andrade, Carlos. *Fazendeiro do ar*. Rio de Janeiro: BestBolso, 2014. (New meeting collection, v. 1.)

Drummond de Andrade, Carlos (1951a). Hotel Toffolo. *In*: Drummond de Andrade, Carlos. *Claro enigma*. Rio de Janeiro: BestBolso, 2014. (New meeting collection, v. 1).

Drummond de Andrade, Carlos (1951b). Tarde de maio. *In*: Drummond de Andrade, Carlos. *Claro enigma*. Rio de Janeiro: BestBolso, 2014. (New meeting collection, v. 1.)

Durban, Joshua. "The very same is lost": in pursuit of mental coverage when emerging from autistic states. *In*: Levine, Howard B.; Power, David G. (org.). *Engaging primitive anxieties of the emerging self: the legacy of Frances Tustin*. London: Karnac, 2017.

Editora Blucher. *Lançamento: Psicanálise e vida covidiana*. YouTube, 2 June, 2021. 1 vídeo (1 h 37 min). Available at: https://www.youtube.com/watch?v=BcoG-RoteRE.

Eekhoff, Judy K. Finding a center of gravity via proximity with the analyst. *In*: Levine, Howard B.; Power, David G. (eds.). *Engaging primitive anxieties of the emerging self: the legacy of Frances Tustin*. London: Karnac, 2017.

Eisenstein, V. W. Differential psychotherapy of borderline states. *Psychiatric Quarterly*, v. 25, pp. 379–401, 1951.

Eissler, Kurt. Remarks on the Psychoanalysis of Schizophrenia. *International Journal of Psychoanalysis*, XXXII, 1951.

Eshel, Ofra. "Black holes" and "fear of breakdown" in the analysis of a fetishistic-masochistic patient. *In*: Levine, Howard B.; Power, David G. (eds.). *Engaging primitive anxieties of the emerging self: the legacy of Frances Tustin*. London: Karnac, 2017.

Fairbairn, William Ronald Dodds. Freud, the psychoanalytical method and mental health. *British Journal of Medical Psychology*, v. 30, part. 2, pp. 53–62, 1957.

Fairbairn, William Ronald Dodds. On the nature and aims of psycho-analytical treatment. *International Journal of Psychoanalysis*, n. 39, pp. 374–385, 1958.

Federn, Paul. The neurotic symptoms in schizophrenia. In: Federn, Paul; Meng, Heinrich (eds.). *Psychoanalytic psychiatry: lectures on application of psychoanalysis to psychiatric disorders*. International Universities Press, 1947, pp. 129–145.

Fenichel, O. (1941). *Problemas de técnica psicoanalítica*. Ciudad de México: Pax México, 1961.

Ferenczi, Sandór (1909). As melodias que vem em nossa mente. *In*: Ferenczi, Sandór. *Sonhos, melodias e sintomas*. Selection of texts and translation by Krüger, Lucas;

Spieler, Eduardo; Gerchman, Felipe. Porto Alegre: Artes & Ecos, 2019. (Série escrita psicanalítica).

Ferenczi, Sándor (1928). A elasticidade da técnica psicanalítica. *In*: Ferenczi, Sandór. *Obras completas de Sandór Ferenczi*. São Paulo: Martins Fontes, 1992. v. 4.

Ferenczi, Sandór (1930). Princípio de relaxamento e neocatarse. *In*: Ferenczi, Sandór. *Obras completas de Sandór Ferenczi*. São Paulo: Martins Fontes, 1992a. v. 4.

Ferenczi, Sandór (1919). Dificuldades técnicas de uma análise de histeria. *In*: Ferenczi, Sandór. *Obras completas de Sándor Ferenczi* (2nd edition). Translated by Álvaro Cabral. São Paulo: WMF Martins Fontes, 2011. v. 3.

Ferenczi, Sándor (1921). Prolongamentos da "técnica ativa" em psicanálise. *In*: Ferenczi, Sandór. *Obras completas de Sándor Ferenczi*. São Paulo: Martins Fontes, 2011a. v. 3.

Ferenczi, Sandór (1931). Análise de crianças com adultos. *In*: Ferenczi, Sandór. *Obras completas de Sandór Ferenczi*. São Paulo: Martins Fontes, 2011b. v. 4.

Ferenczi, Sandór (1915). Inquietude no fim de sessão de análise. *In*: Ferenczi, Sandór. *Sonhos, melodias e sintomas*. Selection of texts and translation by Lucas Krüger, Eduardo Spieler and Felipe Gerchman. Porto Alegre: Artes & Ecos, 2019. (Série escrita psicanalítica.)

Ferro, A. (2009). Transformations in dreaming and characters in the psychoanalytic field. *International Journal of Psychoanalysis*, v. 90, n. 2, pp. 209–230.

Figueiredo, Luís Claudio. A virtualidade do dispositivo de trabalho psicanalítico e o atendimento remoto: uma reflexão em três partes. *Cadernos de Psicanálise*, Rio de Janeiro, v. 42, n. 42, pp. 61–80, January/June, 2020. Available at: http://pepsic.bvsalud.org/pdf/cadpsi/v42n42/v42n42a05.pdf.

Flournoy, Olivier. *Le temps d'une analyse*. Paris: Pierre Belfond, 1979.

Forbes, Jorge. *Da palavra ao gesto do analista*. Text established by Maria Margareth Ferraz de Oliveira. Rio de Janeiro: Jorge Zahar, 1999.

Frank, Claudia (1999). *Melanie Klein in Berlin: her first psychoanalyses of children*. London: Routledge, 2009.

Freud, Sigmund (1915). *O inconsciente: Seção V – As características especiais do sistema Inc*. *In*: Freud, Sigmund. Edição Standard Brasileira das Obras Psicológicas Completas de Sigmund Freud. Translated by Jayme Salomão. Rio de Janeiro: Imago Editora, 1996. v. XIV, pp. 217–222.

Freud, Sigmund. *The standard edition of the complete psychological works of Sigmund Freud*. Translated from the German under the general editorship of James Strachey, in collaboration with Anna Freud. London: Hogarth Press and the Institute of Psycho-Analysis, 1953–1974. 24 v.

Freud, Sigmund (1916). Letter to Andreas-Salome, May 25, 1916. *In*: Pfeiffer, E. (ed.), *Sigmund Freud and Lou Andreas-Salome Letters*. New York: Harcourt, Brace, Jovanovich, 1966.

Freud, Sigmund. *Edição standard brasileira das obras psicológicas completas de Sigmund Freud*. Translated under the direction of Jayme Salomão. Rio de Janeiro: Imago, 1974. 24 v.

Freud, Sigmund (1905 [1904]). Sobre a psicoterapia. *In*: Freud, Sigmund. *Obras psicológicas completas de Sigmund Freud: edição standard brasileira*. Rio de Janeiro: Imago, 1989. v. VII.

Freud, S. *Obras completas*. Rio de Janeiro: Imago, 1996. v. I, II, III.

Freud, Sigmund (1950 [1895]). Projeto para uma psicologia científica. *In*: Freud, Sigmund. *Obras completas*. Rio de Janeiro: Imago, 1996. v. I.

Freud, Sigmund (1895). Psicoterapia da histeria. *In*: Freud, Sigmund. *Obras completas*, Brazilian standard edition. Rio de Janeiro: Imago, 1996a. v. II.

Freud, Sigmund (1896). Análise de um caso de paranóia crônica. *In*: Freud, Sigmund. Observações adicionais sobre as neuropsicoses de defesa. *Obras completas*. Rio de Janeiro: Imago, 1996b. v. III.

Freud, Sigmund (1901). Sobre os sonhos. *In*: Freud, Sigmund. *Obras completas*, Brazilian standard edition. Rio de Janeiro: Imago, 1996c. v. V.

Freud, Sigmund (1912). Recomendações aos médicos que exercem a psicanálise. *In*: Freud, Sigmund. *Obras completas*, Brazilian standard edition. Rio de Janeiro: Imago, 1996d. v. XII.

Freud, Sigmund (1913a). Sobre o início do tratamento (novas recomendações sobre a técnica da psicanálise I). *In*: Freud, Sigmund. *Obras completas*, Brazilian standard edition. Rio de Janeiro: Imago, 1996e. v. XII.

Freud, Sigmund (1914a). Sobre o narcisismo: uma introdução. *In*: Freud, Sigmund. *Obras completas*. Rio de Janeiro: Imago, 1996f. v. XIV.

Freud, Sigmund (1937). Análise terminável e interminável. *In*: Freud, Sigmund. *Obras completas*, Brazilian standard edition. Rio de Janeiro: Imago, 1996g. v. XXIII.

Freud, Sigmund (1908a [1907]). Escritores criativos e devaneios. *In*: Freud, Sigmund. *Obras completas*. Rio de Janeiro: Imago, 2006. v. IX.

Freud, Sigmund (1930). O mal-estar na civilização. *In*: Freud, Sigmund. *Obras completas*. Rio de Janeiro: Imago, 2006a. v. XXI.

Freud, Sigmund (1913b). O início do tratamento. *In*: Freud, Sigmund. *Obras completas*. São Paulo: Companhia das Letras, 2010. v. 10.

Freud, Sigmund (1920). Além do princípio do prazer. *Obras completas*. São Paulo: Companhia das Letras, 2010. v. 14.

Freud, Sigmund. *Obras completas*. Translated by Paulo César de Souza. São Paulo: Companhia das Letras, 2010. 20 v.

Freud, Sigmund (1914b). Recordar, repetir e elaborar. *In*: Freud, Sigmund. *Obras completas*. Translated by Paulo César de Souza. São Paulo: Companhia das Letras, 2010. v. 10.

Freud, Sigmund (1911). Observações psicanalíticas sobre um caso de paranoia (Dementia Paranoides) relatado em autobiografia ("O caso Schreber, 1911"). *In*: Freud, Sigmund. *Obras completas*. Translated by Paulo César de Souza. São Paulo: Companhia das Letras, 2010a. v. 10.

Freud, Sigmund (1918 [1914]). História de uma neurose infantil ("O homem dos lobos"). *In*: Freud, Sigmund. *Obras completas*. São Paulo: Companhia das Letras, 2010b. v. 14.

Freud, Sigmund (1912–1913). Totem e tabu. *In*: Freud, Sigmund. *Obras completas*. Translated by Paulo César de Souza. São Paulo: Companhia das Letras, 2012. v. 11.

Freud, Sigmund (1908b [1907]). O poeta e o fantasiar. *In*: Freud, Sigmund. *Escritos sobre literatura*. Translated by Saulo Krieger. São Paulo: Hedra, 2014.

Freud, Sigmund. Trecho do Manuscrito N, anexo à carta a Fliess, de maio de 1897. *In*: *Obras incompletas de Sigmund Freud*. Translated by Ernani Chaves. Belo Horizonte: Autêntica, 2015.

Freud, Sigmund (1908c [1907]). O poeta e o fantasiar. *In*: Freud, Sigmund. *Obras incompletas de Sigmund Freud*. Translated by Ernani Chaves. Belo Horizonte: Autêntica, 2015a.

Freud, Sigmund (1908d [1907]). O escritor e a fantasia. *In*: Freud, Sigmund. *Obras completas*. Translated by Paulo César de Souza. São Paulo: Companhia das Letras, 2015b. v. VIII.

Freud, Sigmund (1905 [1901]). Análise fragmentária de uma histeria ("O caso Dora"). *In*: Freud, Sigmund. *Obras completas*. São Paulo: Companhia das Letras, 2016. v. 6.

Freud, Sigmund (1905). Três ensaios sobre a teoria da sexualidade. *In*: Freud, Sigmund. *Obras completas*. São Paulo: Companhia das Letras, 2016a. v. 6.

Freud, Sigmund (1900). A interpretação dos sonhos. *In*: Freud, Sigmund. *Obras completas*. Translated by Paulo César de Souza. São Paulo: Companhia das Letras, 2019. v. 4.

Freud, Sigmund (1942 [1905/1906]). Personagens psicopáticos no teatro. *In*: Freud, Sigmund. *Obras completas*. Translation and notes by Paulo César de Souza. São Paulo: Companhia das Letras, 2019a. v. 6.

Friedberg, Ahron; Linn, Louis. The couch as icon. *Psychoanalytic Review*, v. 99, n. 1, pp. 35–62, February, 2012.

Gabbard, Glen O. Technical approaches to transference hate in the analysis of borderline patients. *International Journal of Psychoanalysis*, v. 72, pp. 625–637, 1991.

Gay, Peter. *Freud: uma vida para o nosso tempo*. Translated by Denise Bottman. São Paulo: Companhia das Letras, 1989.

Gedo, John E. Channels of communication and the analytic setup. *Psychoanalytic Inquiry*, v. 15, pp. 294–303, 1995.

Goethe, Johann Wolfgang von. *O jogo das nuvens*. Selection, translation, preface and notes by João Barrento. Porto: Assírio & Alvim, 2003.

Goethe, Johann Wolfgang von. *Fausto: uma tragédia (Part I)*. Translated by Agostinho D'Ornellas. São Paulo: Penguin Classics/Companhia das Letras, 2012.

Goethe, Johann Wolfgang von (1819). *Divã ocidento-oriental*. Translation and afterword by Daniel Martineschen, first edition. São Paulo: Estação Liberdade, 2020. Original title: *West-östlicher divan* (West–Eastern divan).

Goldberger, Marianne (1995). The couch as defense and as potential for enactment. *The Psychoanalytic Quarterly*, v. 64, n. 1, pp. 23–42, 1995.

Grossman, William I. Reflections on a group investigating borderline personality. *In*: Green, André (ed.). *Resonance of suffering countertransference in non-neurotic structures*. London: Karnac, 2007.

Green, André (1977). *Sobre a loucura pessoal*. Tradução de Carlos Alberto Pavanelli. Rio de Janeiro: Imago, 1988.

Green, André. L'enfant modèle. *Nouvelle Revue de Psychanalyse*, n. 19, pp. 27–47, 1979a.

Green, André (1979b). A psicanálise e modos comuns de pensamento. *In*: Green, André. *Sobre a loucura pessoal (coletânea de artigos, 1972–1986)*. Rio de Janeiro: Imago, 1988.

Green, André. *La nueva clínica psicoanalítica y la teoría de Freud: aspectos fundamentales de la locura privada*. Buenos Aires: Amorrortu editores, 1994.

Green, A. (1996). *André Green at the Squiggle Foundation*. Winnicott Studies, 10, 9–23. London: The Squiggle Foundation.

Green, André. The central phobic position: a new formulation of the free association method. *International Journal of Psychoanalysis*, n. 81, pp. 429–451, 2000a.

Green, A. (1988). *Narcisismo de vida, narcisismo de morte*. Translated by Claudia Berliner. São Paulo: Escuta, 2001.

Green, André. The central phobic position: a new formulation of the free association method. *In*: Williams, P. (ed.). *Key papers on borderline disorders*. London: Karnac, 2002.

Green, André (2000b). *André Green e a Fundação Squiggle*. São Paulo: Roca, 2003.

Green, André. O silêncio do psicanalista. *Revista Psychê*, São Paulo, year VIII, n. 14, p. 23, July/December, 2004. Available at: pepsic.bvsalud.org/pdf/psyche/v8n14/v8n14a02.pdf.

Green, André (1986). *A loucura privada*. São Paulo: Escuta, 2005.

Green, André. O enquadre. *In*: Green, André. *Orientações para uma psicanálise contemporânea*. Rio de Janeiro: Imago, 2008.

Green, André. *Orientações para uma psicanálise contemporânea*. Rio de Janeiro: Imago, 2008a.

Green, André. *Illusions and Disillusions of Psychoanalytic Work*. London: Karnac, 2011.

Green, André; Urribarri, Fermando. *Do pensamento clínico ao paradigma contemporâneo: diálogos*. Translated by Paulo Sérgio de Sousa Jr. São Paulo: Blucher, 2019.

Grotstein, James S. A reassessment of the couch in psychoanalysis. *Psychoanalytic Inquiry: A Topical Journal for Mental Health Professionals*, v. 15, n. 3, pp. 396–405, 1995.

Grotstein, James S. (2009) ... *But at the same time and on another level ... clinical applications in the Kleinian/Bionian mode*. London: Karnac, 2009.

Guntrip, Harry (1961). *Personality structure and human interaction: The developing synthesis of psycho-dynamic theory*. New York: International Universities Press, 1964.

Guntrip, Harry. *Schizoid phenomena object-relations and the self*. New York: International Universities Press, 1969.

Hafez. 2019. *The divan of Hafez: a bilingual edition, poems from the Persian*. Translated by Reza Saberi. Bethesda, MD: Ibex Publishers.

Hanns, Luiz Alberto. A atualidade de Freud e um novo modo de traduzi-lo. *In*: Tavares, Pedro Heliodoro (ed.). *Psicanálise entre línguas*. Rio de Janeiro: 7 Letras, 2016.

Heimann, Paula. (1958). Notes on early development. In: Heimann, P.; Tonnesmann, M. (Eds.). *Children no longer: Collected papers of Paula Heimann, 1949–1980*. Routledge, 2025.

Heimann, P. (1975a). Further observations on the analyst's cognitive process. In: Heimann, P.; Tonnesmann, M. (Eds.). *Children no longer: Collected papers of Paula Heimann, 1949–1980*. Routledge, 2025.

Heimann, Paula (1975b). Sacrificial parapraxis – failure or achievement? *In*: Heimann, Paula. *About children and children no longer: Collected papers 1942–1980*. London; New York: Routledge, 2005a.

Hopkins, Linda. *False self: the life of Masud Khan*. London: Karnac, 2008.

Houzel, Didier. Precipitation anxiety in the analysis of adult patients. *In*: Mitrani, Judith L.; Mitrani, Theodore (eds.). *Frances Tustin today*. New York: Routledge, 2015.

Huidobro, Vicente. *Arte póetica*. *In*: Huidobro, Vicente. *El espejo de agua*. Buenos Aires: Órion, 1916.

Isaacs, Susan (1952). The nature and function of phantasy. *In*: Klein, Melanie; Heimann, Paula; Isaacs, Susan; Riviere, Joan (eds.). *Developments in psychoanalysis*. London: Karnac, 2002.

Jaber, Maíra dos Santos. *O bebê e a música*: sobre a percepção e a estruturação do estímulo musical, do pré-natal ao segundo ano de vida pós-natal. Dissertation (Master's degree in Music, School of Music, Postgraduate Program in Music, Universidade Federal do Rio de Janeiro, Rio de Janeiro, 2013. Available at: http://objdig.ufrj.br/26/dissert/817223.pdf.

Jacobson, Jacob G. The analytic couch: Facilitator or sine qua non? *Psychoanalytic Inquiry*, v. 15, 1995.

Jorge, Marco Antonio Coutinho. *Fundamentos da psicanálise de Freud a Lacan*. A prática analítica, first edition. Rio de Janeiro: Zahar, 2017. v. 3.

Junqueira de Mattos, José Américo. Impressions of my analysis with Dr. Bion. *In*: Levine, Howard B.; Civitarese, Giuseppe. *The W. R. Bion tradition: lines of development – evolution of theory and practice over the decades*. London: Routledge, 2016.

Kahn, Laurence. Se apenas soubéssemos o que existe! *In*: Levine, Howard B.; Reed, Gail S.; Scarfone, Dominique (eds.). *Estados não representados e a construção de significado: contribuições clínicas e teóricas*. São Paulo: Blucher, 2016.

Khan, M. Masud Raza. *The privacy of the self: papers on psychoanalytic theory and technique*. London: Karnac, 1996.
Kelmon, Harold. The use of the analytic couch. *American Journal of Psychoanalysis*, v. 14, n. 1, 1954.
Klein, George S. *Perception, motives, and personality*. New York: Knopf, 1970.
Klein, Melanie (1957). Inveja e gratidão. *In*: *Obras completas de Melanie Klein: inveja e gratidão e outros trabalhos (1946–1963)*. Rio de Janeiro: Imago, 1991. v. III.
Klein, Melanie. Narrativa da análise de um a criança; o procedimento da psicanálise de crianças tal como observado no tratamento de um menino de dez anos. *In*: Klein, Melanie. *Obras completas de Melanie Klein*. Rio de Janeiro: Imago, 1994. v. IV.
Klein, Melanie (1932). A técnica da análise no período de latência. *In*: Klein, Melanie. *Obras completas de Melanie Klein: a psicanálise de crianças*. Rio de Janeiro: Imago, 1997. v. II. Original title (1999): Melanie Kleins erste Kinderanalysen: die Entdeckung des Kindes als Objekt sui generis von Heilen und Forschen.
Klein, Sydney. Autistic phenomena in neurotic patients. *In*: Mitrani, Judith L.; Mitrani, Theodore (eds.). *Frances Tustin today*. New York: Routledge, 2015.
Korbivcher, Celia F. Bion and the unintegrated states: falling, dissolving, and spilling. *In*: Levine, Howard B.; Power, David G. (eds.). *Engaging primitive anxieties of the emerging self: the legacy of Frances Tustin*. London: Karnac, 2017.
Kris, Anton O. *Free association: method and process*. Hillsdale, NJ: Analytic Press, 1996.
Krüger, Lucas. Sonoridades clínicas. *In*: Krüger, Lucas; Refosco, Lísia da Luz; Silva, Sander Machado da (eds.). *Interlocuções na fronteira entre psicanálise e arte*. Porto Alegre: Artes & Ecos, 2017.
Krüger, Lucas. *Homenagem à nuvem*. Artes & Ecos: Porto Alegre, 2017a.
Krüger, Lucas. Rá. *In*: Krüger, Lucas. *Homenagem à nuvem*. Artes & Ecos, 2017b.
Krüger, Lucas. A poesia, a escuta, e o uso da palavra na clínica psicanalítica. *In*: Krüger, Lucas; Refosco, Lísia da Luz; Silva, Sander Machado da (eds.). *Interlocuções na fronteira entre psicanálise e arte*. Porto Alegre: Artes & Ecos, 2017c.
Krüger, Lucas. Sobre as reflexões de Christopher Bollas a respeito do fascismo e do genocídio. *Sig revista de psicanálise*, Porto Alegre, v. 10, n. 18, p. 31–40, jan./jun. 2021.
Krüger, Lucas. A necessidade do divã ou um substituto que não o olhar. *In*: Kupermann, D.; Gondar, J.; Dal Molin, E.C. (eds.). *Ferenczi: pensador da catástrofe*. São Paulo: Zagodoni, 2022.
Kupermann, Daniel. *Por que Ferenczi?* São Paulo: Zagodoni, 2019.
Kupermann, Daniel. *Presença sensível: cuidado e criação na clínica psicanalítica*. Porto Alegre: Artes & Ecos, 2021.
Kupermann, D.; Gondar, J.; Dal Molin, E.C. *Ferenczi: pensador da catástrofe*. São Paulo: Zagodoni, 2022.
Lable, Ira; Kelley, John M.; Ackerman, Julie; Levy, Raymond; Waldron, Sherwood Jr.; Ablon, J. Stuart. The role of the couch in psychoanalysis: proposed research designs and some preliminary data. *Journal of the American Psychoanalytic Association*, v. 58, n. 5, pp. 861–887, October, 2010. Available at: citeseerx.ist.psu.edu/viewdoc/downloaddoi=10.1.1.1033.9718&rep=rep1&type=pdf.
Lacan, Jacques (1954–1955). *O Seminário, livro 2: o eu na teoria de Freud e na técnica da psicanálise*. Rio de Janeiro: Zahar, 1995.
Lacan, Jacques (1955–1956). *O Seminário, livro 3: as psicoses*. Rio de Janeiro: Zahar, 1997.
Lacan, Jacques (1955). A coisa freudiana: ou sentido do retorno a Freud em psicanálise. *In*: Lacan, Jacques. *Escritos*. Rio de Janeiro: Jorge Zahar, 1998.

Lacan, Jacques (1958) A direção do tratamento e os princípios de seu poder. *In*: *Escritos*. Translated by Vera Ribeiro. Rio de Janeiro: Zahar, 1998.

Lacan, Jacques (1975–1976). *O Seminário, livro 23: o sinthoma*. Rio de Janeiro: Zahar, 2007.

Laplanche, Jean. *Vida e morte em psicanálise*. Translated by Cleonice Paes Barreto Mourão e Consuelo Fortes Santiago. Porto Alegre: Artes Médicas, 1985.

Laplanche, Jean (1987). *A Tina: a transcendência da transferência*. São Paulo: Martins Fontes, 1993.

Lewin, D. Bertram. Dream psychology and the analytic situation. *Psychoanalytic Quarterly*, v. 24, n. 2, 1955.

Little, Margaret I. (1990). *Ansiedades psicóticas e prevenção: registro pessoal de uma análise com Winnicott*. Rio de Janeiro: Imago, 1992.

Lora, Débora Zaffari; Paim Filho, Ignácio A.; Nunes, Luciana Nunes de. Percepção – castração – cisão: as múltiplas faces do Eu. *Revistas do CEPdePA*, v. 25, 2018. Available at: http://www.cepdepa.com.br/wp-content/uploads/2020/02/5-Percep%C3%A7%C3%A3o-%E2%80%93-castra%-C3%A7%C3%A3o-%E2%80%93-cis%C3%A3o-as-m%C3%Baltiplas-faces-do-Eu.pdf

Lutenberg, Jaime M. Mental void and the borderline patient. *In*: Green, André (ed.). *Resonance of suffering countertransference in non-neurotic structures*. London: Karnac, 2007.

Macalpine, Ida. The development of the transference. *Psychoanalytic Quarterly*, v. 19, n. 4, pp. 501–539, 1950.

Mayakovski, Vladimir. A nuvem de calças. *In*: Blok, Aleksandr et al. *Poetas Russos*. Translation, prologue and notes by Manuel de Seabra. Lisbon: Relógio D' Água Editores, 1995.

Mannoni, Maud. O divã de Procusto. *In*: McDougall, Joyce (coordinator). *O divã de Procusto*. Porto Alegre: Artes Médicas, 1991.

Marucco, Norberto. O analisando de hoje e o inconsciente (sobre o conceito de zonas psíquicas). *Revista de Psicanálise da SPPA*, v. 10, n. 3, pp. 453–473, 2003.

Marucco, Norberto. A clínica contemporânea e suas raízes metapsicoló-gicas freudianas. *Jornal de Psicanálise*, São Paulo, v. 45, n. 83, December, 2012.

Marucco, Norberto. A prática psicanalítica contemporânea: as zonas psí-quicas e os processos de insconscientização. *Revista de Psicanálise*, v. 15, n. 1, pp. 133–136, 2013.

Mattuella, Luciano. *O corpo do analista*. Porto Alegre: Artes & Ecos, 2020. (Série escrita psicanalítica.)

McDougall, Joyce (1982). *Teatros do eu*. Rio de Janeiro: Francisco Alves, 1989.

McDougall, Joyce (1989). *Teatros do corpo*. São Paulo: Martins Fontes, 1996.

McLaughlin, James T. Nonverbal behaviors in the analytic situation: the search for meaning in nonverbal cues. *In*: Kramer, Selma; Akhtar, Salman (eds.). *When the body speaks: psychological meanings in kinetic clues*. Northvale, NJ: Aronson, 1992.

Mélega, Marisa Pelella. *Post-autism: a psychoanalytical narrative with supervisions by Donald Meltzer*. London: Karnac, 2014.

Meltzer, Donald. *The claustrum: an investigation of claustrophobic phenomena. Strath Tag, Perthshire*, Scotland: The Clunie Press, 1992a. (The Roland Harris Trust Library, 15.)

Meltzer, Donald. *Sincerity and other works: collected papers of Donald Meltzer*. London: Karnac, 1994.

Meltzer, D. (1992b). *The claustrum: an investigation of claustrophobic phenomena*. London: Karnac, 2008.

Meltzer, Donald (1984). *Dream-life: a re-examination of the psychoanalytic theory and technique*. London: Karnac, 2009.

Meltzer, Donald; Harris, Martha. *Adolescence: talks and papers by Donald Meltzer and Martha Harris*. Edited by Martha Harris. London: Karnac, 2011.

Meltzer, Donald (1967). *The psycho-analytical process*. London: Karnac, 2018.

Mendes, Murilo (1930). *Poemas*. São Paulo: Cosac Naify, 2014.

Mendes, Murilo (1944). *Metamorfoses*. São Paulo: Cosac Naify, 2015.

Miller, Gérard (director.). Rendez-vous chez Lacan. [Documentary.] France: PMP; 2 Cafés l'Addition, 2011. 52 min.

Milner, Marion (1948). Um paciente adulto utiliza brinquedos. *In*: MILNER, Marion. *A loucura suprimida do homem são: quarenta e quatro anos explorando a psicanálise*. Translated by Paulo Cesar Sandler. Rio de Janeiro: Imago, 1991.

Milton, Christopher. *A phenomenological hermeneutic investigation into the psychoanalytic psychotherapist's experience of using the psychoanalytic couch*. 2003. Thesis (Doctoral), Rhodes University, Grahamstown, 2004.

Mitrani, Judith L. Trying to enter the long black branches: Some technical extensions for the analysis of autistic states in adults. *In*: Mitrani, Judith L.; Mitrani, Theodore (eds.). *Frances Tustin today*. New York: Routledge, 2015.

Mitrani, Judith L.; Mitrani, Theodore. *Frances Tustin today*. New York: Routledge, 2015.

Money-Kyrle, Roger E. Introdução a amor, culpa e reparação. *In*: Klein, Melanie (1921–1945). *Obras completas de Melanie Klein*. Rio de Janeiro: Imago, 1996. v. I.

Nasio, Juan David. *O olhar em psicanálise*. Rio de Janeiro: Jorge Zahar, 1995.

Neruda, Pablo. *El libro de las preguntas*. Buenos Aires: Editorial Losada, 1974.

Ogden, Thomas. The structure of experience. *In*: Ogden, Thomas. *The primitive edge of experience*. New Jersey: Jason Aronson, 1989.

Ogden, Thomas. The autistic-contiguous position. *In*: Ogden, Thomas. *The primitive edge of experience*. New Jersey: Jason Aronson, 1989a.

Ogden, Thomas. *Subjects of analysis*. New Jersey: Jason Aronson, 1994.

Ogden, Thomas. *Conversations at the frontier of dreaming*. London: Karnac, 2002.

Ogden, Thomas. Re-minding the body. *In*: Ogden, Thomas. *Conversations at the frontier of dreaming*. London: Karnac, 2002a.

Ogden, Thomas. *His art of psychoanalyis: dreaming undreamt dreams and interrupted cries*. New York: Routledge, 2005a.

Ogden, Thomas (2005b). Sobre sustentar e conter, ser e sonhar. *In*: Ogden, Thomas. *Esta arte da psicanálise: sonhando sonhos não sonhados e gritos interrompidos*. Porto Alegre: Artmed, 2010.

Ogden, Thomas. Privacidade, reverie e técnica analítica. *In*: Ogden, Thomas. *Reverie e interpretação: captando algo humano*. São Paulo: Escuta, 2013.

Ogden, Thomas. *Leituras criativas: ensaios sobre obras analíticas seminais*. São Paulo: Escuta, 2014.

Ogden, Thomas. *Reclaiming unlived life: experiences in psychoanalysis*. New York; London: Routledge, 2016.

Oliveira, Ana Lúcia Monteiro. Poltrona elástica? Divã transicional? Reflexões sobre a minha poltrona giratória. *Revista da SPPA*, Porto Alegre, v. 27, n. 2, 2020.

Pontalis, Jean-Bertrand. *Entre o sonho e a dor*. Aparecida, SP: Ideias & Letras, 2005.

Pontalis, Jean-Bertrand. Na borda das palavras. [Interview given to] Marcelo Marques. *Percurso*, October, 2008. Available at: https://www.revistapercurso.com.br/index.php?apg=artigo_view&ida=40&ori=entrev#topo.

Pound, Ezra. *ABC da literatura*. São Paulo: Cultrix, 2013.

Quinet, Antonio. *As 4+1 condições da análise*, twelfth editiond. Rio de Janeiro: Jorge Zahar, 2009.

Quinodoz, Danielle. *Words that touch: a psychoanalyst learns to speak*. London: Karnac, 2003.

Rank, Otto. *O trauma do nascimento: e seu significado para a psicanálise. Translation and introduction by Érica Gonçalves de Castro*. São Paulo: Cienbook, 2016.

Rriolfi, Claudia. Quando está indicado o divã: a análise lacaniana tem contraindicações? *In*: Riolfi, Claudia; Forbes, Jorge (eds.). *Psicanálise: a clínica do real*. Barueri: Manole. Digital edition, 2014.

Rose, Gilbert J. Unconscious birth fantasies in the ninth month of treatment. *Journal of the American Psychoanalytic Association*, v. 10, pp. 677–688, 1962.

Rosen, V. The nature of verbal interventions in psychoanalysis. *Psychoanalysis and Contemporary Science*, v. 3, pp. 189–209, 1974.

Ross, John Munder. Once more onto the couch: consciousness and preconscious defenses in the psychoanalytic situation and process. *Journal of the American Psychoanalytic Association*, v. 47, n. 1, p. 99, 1999.

Roudinesco, Élisabeth. Élisabeth Roudinesco: Freud nos tornou heróis da nossa vida. [Interview given to A. V.]. *El país*, 6 September, 2015. Cultura. Available at: brasil.elpais.com/brasil/2015/09/02/cultura/1441210297_491115.html.

Roussillon, René (2005). A conversão psicanalítica: um divã em latência. Translation by Eline Batistella. Available at: https://issuu.com/psicossomaticainstitutosedessapient/docs/a_conversacao_psicanalitica_por_r_roussillon. Original: La «conversation» psychanalytique: un divan en latence. *Revue Française de Psychanalyse*, v. 69, pp. 365–381, 2005/2.

Roussillon, René. *Primitive agony and symbolization*. London: Karnac, 2011.

Roussillon, René. Satisfaction et plaisir partagé. *Revue française de psychanalyse*, France, v. 74, pp. 21–38, 2010.

Roussillon, René. The function of the object in the binding and unbinding of the drives. *International Journal of Psychoanalysis*, v. 94, pp. 257–276, 2013.

Roussillon, René. *Le transitionnel, le sexuel et la réflexivité*. Paris: Dunod, 2008.

Roussillon, René. Aspects métapsychologiques des médiations thérapeutiques. *Cliniques*, n. 12, pp. 230–245, 2016/2.

Roussillon, Le transitionnel et le travail psychanalytique en séance. *Revue française de psychanalyse*, v. 82, pp. 121–131, 2018/1.

Roussillon, René. *Manual da prática clínica em psicologia e psicopatologia*. São Paulo: Blucher, 2019.

Sadow, L. Looking, listening, and the couch. *Psychoanalytic Inquiry*, v. 15, n. 3, pp. 386–395, 1995.

Salomão, Waly (1996). Poema Jet-lagged. *In*: Salomão, Waly. *Algaravias: Câmara de ecos. Poesia Total*. São Paulo: Companhia das Letras, 2014.

Santos, Guilherme Geha dos; Mello Neto, Gustavo Adolfo Ramos. Pacientes, problemas e fronteiras: psicanálise e quadros borderline. *Psicologia USP*, São Paulo, v. 29, n. 2, pp. 285–293, May–August, 2018. Available at: http://dx.doi.org/10.1590/0103-656420170101.

Schachter, Joseph; Kächele, Horst. The couch in psychoanalysis. *Contemporary Psychoanalysis*, v. 46, n. 3, pp. 439–459, 2010.

Schermer, Victor L. *Meaning, mind, and self-transformation: psychoanalytic interpretation and the interpretation of psychoanalysis*. London: Karnac, 2014.

Schmideberg, Melitta. A note on claustrophobia. *Psychoanalytic Review*, n. 35, pp. 309–311, 1948.

Searles, Harold F. *The nonhuman environment in normal development and in schizophrenia*. New York: International Universities Press, 1960.

Searles, Harold F. (1976). Transitional phenomena and therapeutic symbiosis. *In*: *Countertransference and related subjects*. Madison, CT: International Universities Press, 1979. pp. 503–576.

Segal, H. (1950). Some aspects of the analysis of a schizophrenic. *In*: *The work of Hanna Segal: a Kleinian approach to clinical practice*. New York: Jason Aronson, 1981.

Segal, H. (1956). Depression in the schizophrenic. *In*: *The work of Hanna Segal: a Kleinian approach to clinical practice*. New York: Jason Aronson, 1981.

Segal, Naomi. *Consensuality: Didier Anzieu, gender and the sense of touch*. Amsterdam/New York: Rodopi, 2009.

Shelley, Percy (1840 [1815]). Uma defesa da poesia. *In*: Shelley, Percy. *Uma defesa da poesia e outros ensaios*. São Paulo: Landmark, 2008.

Simmel, Ernst (1943). *A autoconservação e a pulsão de morte*. Ttanslation and introduction by Gabriel K. Saito. Porto Alegre: Artes & Ecos, 2022. (Série escrita psicanalítica.)

Skolnick, Neil J. Rethinking the use of the couch: a relational perspective. *Contemporary Psychoanalysis*, v. 51, n. 4, pp. 624–648, 2015.

Souza, Jovelina M. R. de. As origens da noção de poíesis. *Revista Hypnos*, São Paulo, year 13, n. 19, pp. 85–962, second semester, 2007.

Spielrein, Sabina (1912). *A destruição como origem do devir*. Translation by Renata Dias Mundt. Curatorship and introduction by Renata Udler Cromberg. Porto Alegre: Artes & Ecos, 2021. (Série escrita psicanalítica.)

Staehle, Angelika. The threatening character of change: an approach with patients who experience progress as trauma. *In*: Levine, Howard B.; Brown, J. Lawrence (eds.). *Growth and turbulence in the container/ contained: Bion's continuing legacy*. London: Routledge, 2013.

Stein, Martin H. States of consciousness in the analytic situation: including a note on the traumatic dream. *In*: Schur, M. (ed.). *Drives, affects, behavior*, New York: International Universities Press, 1965. v. 2.

Stern, Adolph. Psychoanalytic therapy in the borderline neuroses. *Psychoanalytic Quarterly*, v. 14, n. 2, pp. 190–198, 1945.

Strand, Mark. *Collected poems of Mark Strand*. New York: Knopf, 2016.

Szymborska, Wisława. *Poemas*. Translation by Regina Przybycien. São Paulo: Companhia das Letras, 2011.

Tustin, Frances. *Autistic barriers in neurotic patients*. London: Karnac, 1986.

Tustin, Frances. *Autism and childhood psychosis*. London: Karnac, 1995.

Urribarri, Fernando. André Green: paixão clínica, pensamento complexo. Em direção ao futuro da psicanálise. *Contemporânea – Revista de Psicanálise e Transdisciplinaridade*, Porto Alegre, n. 10, p. 40, July/December, 2010. Available at: www.revistacontemporanea.org.br/revistacontemporaneaanterior/site/wp-content/artigos/AndreGreen.pdf.

Urribarri, Fernando. Os casos-limite e a psicanálise contemporânea: do desafio clínico à complexidade teórica. Interview with André Green. *Sig Revista de Psicanálise*, Porto Alegre, v. 1, n. 2, January–June, 2013.

Valéry, Paul (1937/1938). O ensino da poética no Collège de France. *In*: Valéry, Paul. *Lições de poética*. Belo Horizonte: Âyiné, 2018.

Waugaman, Richard M. The analytic couch as transference object. *Psychoanalytic Inquiry: A Topical Journal for Mental Health Professionals*, v. 15, n. 3, pp. 338–357, 1995.

Winnicott, Donald Woods. *Playing and reality*. London: Tavistock Publications, 1971a.

Winnicott, Donald Woods. *O brincar e a realidade*. Rio de Janeiro: Imago, 1975.

Winnicott, Donald Woods (1953). Objetos transicionais e fenômenos transicionais. *In*: *O brincar e a realidade*. Rio de Janeiro: Imago, 1975a.

Winnicott, Donald Woods (1967). O papel de espelho da mãe e da família no desenvolvimento infantil. *In*: Winnicott, Donald Woods. *O brincar e a realidade*. Rio de Janeiro: Imago, 1975b.

Winnicott, Donald Woods (1969). A localização da experiência cultural. *In*: Winnicott, Donald Woods. *O brincar e a realidade*. Rio de Janeiro: Imago, 1975c.

Winnicott, Donald Woods (1971b). O lugar em que vivemos. *In*: *O brincar e a realidade*. Rio de Janeiro: Imago, 1975d.

Winnicott, Donald Woods (1945a). O desenvolvimento emocional primário. *In*: Winnicott, Donald Woods. *Da pediatria à psicanálise: obras escolhidas*. Porto Alegre: Artes Médicas, 1982.

Winnicott, Donald Woods (1945b). *Da pediatria à psicanálise: obras escolhidas*. Porto Alegre: Artes Médicas, 1982.

Winnicott, Donald Woods (1962). Os objetivos do tratamento psicanalítico. *In*: Winnicott, Donald Woods. *O ambiente e os processos de maturação: estudos sobre a teoria do desenvolvimento emocional*. Porto Alegre: Artes Médicas, 1984.

Winnicott, Donald Woods (1971c). *Consultas terapêuticas em psiquiatria infantil*. Translation by Joseti Marques Xisto Cunha. Rio de Janeiro: Imago, 1984a.

Winnicott, Donald Woods (1972). *Holding and interpretation: fragment of an analysis*. London: The Hogarth Press, 1986.

Winnicott, Donald Woods (1954a). Retraimento e regressão. *In*: *Da pediatria à psicanálise: obras escolhidas*. Rio de Janeiro: Francisco Alves, 1993.

Winnicott, Donald Woods (1964–1968). O jogo do rabisco [Squiggle Game]. *In*: Winnicott, Clare; Shepherd, Ray; Davis, Madeleine (eds.). *Explorações psicanalíticas: D. W. Winnicott*. Porto Alegre: Artmed, 1994.

Winnicott, Donald Woods (1947). O ódio na contratransferência. *In*: Winnicott, Donald Woods. *Da pediatria à psicanálise: obras escolhidas*. Rio de Janeiro: Imago, 2000.

Winnicott, Donald Woods (1954b). Retraimento e regressão. *In*: Winnicott, Donald Woods. *Da pediatria à psicanálise: obras escolhidas*. Rio de Janeiro: Imago, 2000a.

Winnicott, Donald Woods. *O brincar e a realidade*. São Paulo: Ubu Editora, 2019.

Wolf, Ernest S. Brief notes on using the couch. *Psychoanalytic Inquiry*, v. 15, pp. 314–323, 1995.

Index

For Product Safety Concerns and Information please contact our EU representative GPSR@taylorandfrancis.com
Taylor & Francis Verlag GmbH, Kaufingerstraße 24, 80331 München, Germany

www.ingramcontent.com/pod-product-compliance
Ingram Content Group UK Ltd.
Pitfield, Milton Keynes, MK11 3LW, UK
UKHW020009200926
475702UK00015B/2557
* 9 7 8 1 0 4 1 1 5 7 9 3 9 *